Glossary 4

Introduction 7

Definitions: diagnosis and comorbidity 11

Etiology 20

Epidemiology 32

The patient's perspective 37

Enhanced care 47

Short-term treatments 55

Long-term treatments 71

The future 88

Useful resources 91

Disclosure 93

Appendix: Generic and brand names of drugs 95

Index 97

Glossary

Antipsychotic drugs: medicines that are primarily used to treat psychotic symptoms. Typical antipsychotics, of which the prototype was chlorpromazine, readily produce motor side effects – usually restlessness or rigidity. They are also sometimes called neuroleptics or major tranquilizers. Atypical antipsychotics have been developed in recent years to reduce the motor side-effect burden. Antipsychotics all antagonize the actions of the neurotransmitter dopamine, and are also antimanic.

Axis I: in the recommended diagnostic scheme of the *Diagnostic and Statistical Manual of Mental Disorders*, Fourth edition (DSM-IV), illnesses are classified on separate axes, which are independent of each other (as, for example, shape and color might be). Axis I diagnoses are the primary psychiatric disorders like bipolar I disorder or schizophrenia.

Axis II: this other axis of the DSM-IV scheme classifies patients according to lifelong personality characteristics if these are judged to be extreme – the so-called personality disorders. Personality diagnoses are not very reliable, but they capture something important about extreme personality styles.

Bipolar: this term is used to describe a range of illnesses in which there are disturbances of mood into both depression and elation – the poles of affective experience.

Bipolar I disorder: a diagnosis that requires simply a single episode of mania. However, it is the rule that patients who experience mania also experience major depression.

Bipolar II disorder: a diagnosis that requires a history of both hypomania and major depression.

Cognitive–behavior therapy (CBT): a psychological treatment that derives from the idea that conscious thoughts and explicit beliefs may exacerbate mood or anxiety states. The therapy aims to elicit and question such thoughts and beliefs and to challenge patients to behave differently when they have them. It has a strong tradition of empirical measurement and a much better evidence base than most 'talking therapies' or 'counseling'.

Cognitive impairment: human cognition can be thought of as a collection of different domains such as attention, memory and executive function. Performance in these different domains can be measured more or less independently and compared with the average for individuals of a given age and education. A person is said to show cognitive impairment when they perform poorly in one or more of these domains. Even small impairments are of interest because they predict difficulty at work, especially for able people.

***Diagnostic and Statistical Manual of Mental Disorders*, Fourth edition (DSM-IV):** published by the American Psychiatric Association, DSM-IV lays out simple rules for making psychiatric diagnosis which enable diagnostic reliability to be achieved. These rules – and hence the diagnostic categories – are, however, arbitrary. They should be thought of as working hypotheses (and may turn out to be false), but they provide an essential preliminary framework for scientific psychiatry.

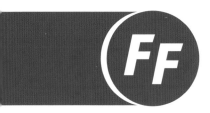

FAST FACTS

Bipolar Disorder

Indispensable
Guides to
Clinical
Practice

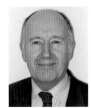

Guy Goodwin DPhil FRCPsych
Professor of Psychiatry
University of Oxford Department of Psychiatry
Warneford Hospital
Oxford, UK

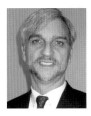

Gary Sachs MD
Director of Harvard Bipolar Research Program and
Associate Professor of Psychiatry
Harvard Medical School
Boston, USA

This book is as balanced and as practical as we can make it. Ideas for
improvements are always welcome: feedback@fastfacts.com

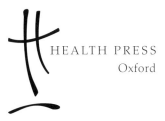

HEALTH PRESS
Oxford

Fast Facts – Bipolar Disorder
First published February 2004

Text © 2004 Guy Goodwin, Gary Sachs

© 2004 in this edition Health Press Limited
Health Press Limited, Elizabeth House, Queen Street, Abingdon,
Oxford OX14 3JR, UK
Tel: +44 (0)1235 523233
Fax: +44 (0)1235 523238

Book orders can be placed by telephone or via the website.
For regional distributors or to order via the website, please go to:
www.fastfacts.com
For telephone orders, please call 01752 202301 (UK) or
800 538 1287 (North America, toll free).

Fast Facts is a trademark of Health Press Limited.

A CIP catalogue record for this title is available from the British Library.

ISBN 1-903734-50-9

Author Goodwin (Guy)
Fast Facts – Bipolar Disorder/
Guy Goodwin, Gary Sachs

The cover shows a functional MRI image of activation in the
ventral striatum during reward. By courtesy of Dr Robert Rogers.

Medical illustrations by Dee McLean, London, UK.
Typesetting and page layout by Zed, Oxford, UK.
Printed by Fine Print (Services) Ltd, Oxford, UK.

Printed with vegetable inks on fully biodegradable and
recyclable paper manufactured from sustainable forests.

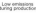
Low emissions
during production

Low
chlorine

Sustainable
forests

panic disorder 16, 52
paranoia 14
paroxetine 65, 95
patient education 47–8
  carbamazepine 87
  lamotrigine 87
  lithium 86
  valproate 86
patients, impact on 8, 33, 35, 37–46
personality characteristics/disorders 4, 18
pharmacogenetics 88
pharmacokinetics 5
phenelzine 65, 95
physical harm 11
pituitary gland 5
placebo 5, 63, 73
placebo-controlled trials 58, 59, 60, 67, 68, 71, 74
positron emission tomography 30
predictability 13
pregnancy and prescribing 63, 77–9, 80
prevalence 8
primary care physicians 9, 32, 51
primary psychiatric disorders 4
  see also bipolar I; schizophrenia; and others by name
psychiatrists 9, 14, 32, 34, 51
psychological interventions 8
psychomotor agitation 12, 15
psychomotor retardation 14, 15, 18
psychopharmacology 25–6, 89
  depression 25–6
  mania 24–5
  see also BAP 55, 56
psychosis 5, 7, 18, 20, 21, 22, 29
  see also drug-induced
psychotic exhaustion 11
psychotropic medicines 5, 27, 58

quetiapine 57, 59, 61, 68, 77, 95

randomized controlled trials 5, 9, 61, 73

rapid cycling 16, 27, 67, 72, 74
  ultrarapid 19
reality, loss of contact with 5
recovery 8, 55
relapse 47, 49, 53, 66, 71, 74, 76, 77, 78, 79
  prevention strategies 72, 73, 75
relationship difficulties 18
reliability of diagnosis 11
research agenda 9, 90
respect for patient 46
restlessness 4, 5, 15
rigidity 4
risperidone 57, 59, 61, 68, 77, 95

safety information (drugs) 81
schizo-affective states 13, 20
schizophrenia 4, 7, 8, 13, 20, 21, 22, 23, 24, 29, 58, 60, 74, 77
scientific approach 37–9, 44, 45, 88
secondary mania 17
seizures as treatment 5
selective serotonin reuptake inhibitors (SSRIs) 26, 64, 65, 67, 69
self-harm 18, 32
  see also suicidal inclinations
self-monitoring 49, 53
sense of control 49
serotonin 25–6, 29
sertraline 65, 95
services, failure of 8
short-term treatments 55–70
side effects 51
  chlorpromazine 4
  see also adverse effects
skills 47, 48–9, 53
sleep disturbance 28, 29, 48–9, 62
social harm 11
social withdrawal 8
spectroscopy 30
stiffness/slowing 5
stigma of psychiatric illness 42–6
stimulants 18, 34–5
substance misuse 16–17, 18, 32, 42, 49, 53, 77
substrate depletion 24–6

suicidal inclinations/ideation 7, 13, 14, 15, 18, 37, 71, 76, 78
  assessment 64
  switching 67, 69
  see also rapid cycling
symptoms
  chronic 55
  major depression 14, 15, mania 11, 12
  remission 68, 69

talking therapies 4
tardive dyskinesia 6, 60, 74, 76
terminology and stigma 44–6
therapeutic alliance/relationship 47
therapists 9
thyroid disease 17
  see also hyperthyroidism; hypothyroidism
thyrotropin 27
thyrotropin-releasing hormone 27
thyroxine 28
topiramate 61, 71, 95
tranquilizers, major 4, 58
tranylcypromine 63, 65, 95
treatment 47, 84–5, 88, 89–90
  see also acute; long-term; short-term
tricyclic antidepressants (TCAs) 63–5, 67, 69
triggers 23, 28, 67

unipolar disorder 6, 7, 14, 18, 20, 21, 26, 29, 32, 33, 35, 63
upward staring 5
useful resources 91–2

valproate 56, 57, 59, 60–1, 62, 65, 66, 68, 69, 72, 73, 75, 76, 78, 80, 82, 84, 86, 95
  in pregnancy 77, 78–9

weight gain 51, 76
weight loss 15
worthlessness 15

Young Mania Rating Scale (YMRS) 59, 60
young patients 33–6

ziprasidone 57, 59, 68, 95

Electroconvulsive therapy (ECT): a very effective treatment for severe depression and, probably, for mania. Before the introduction of ECT in the 1930s, the induction of seizures to treat psychosis was performed chemically. The use of electricity was, and to some extent still is, highly controversial. It is now extremely safe when performed under brief general anesthesia together with a neuromuscular blocker to prevent musculoskeletal damage. The main disadvantage is its effects on memory. Some of the complaints made about ECT are, however, so extreme that they should be viewed as unexplained medical symptoms.

Endogenous: originating from within the body.

Exogenous: having its origins from without (cf: endogenous).

Extrapyramidal side effects (EPS): antipsychotics block dopamine neurotransmission in the basal ganglia of the brain, which leads to EPS. Acute effects include motor restlessness (akathisia), stiffness/slowing and gait disturbance. These symptoms resemble those seen in Parkinson's disease – a degenerative disease of the dopamine neurons in the basal ganglia. More rarely, antipsychotics may also provoke acute dystonic reactions – abnormal postures often accompanied by upward staring of the eyes.

Hypomania: characterized by the presence of mood elevation, usually resulting in increased energy and confidence but without impairment of function (indeed, often the converse – improved attainment).

Hypothalamic–pituitary–adrenal (HPA) axis: the secretion of cortisol from the cortex of the adrenal gland is controlled by adrenocorticotropic hormone from the pituitary gland at the base of the brain and this, in turn, is controlled by corticotropin-releasing hormone secreted into the portal pituitary system in the hypothalamus.

Mania: a mental state of extreme mood elevation or irritability which is accompanied by characteristic changes in behavior and impairment of normal personal or social function. There may be associated psychotic features.

Pharmacokinetic: effects on drug action caused by changes in drug availability (or drug levels) – for example, because of changes in drug metabolism or absorption.

Placebo: inert tablets that are matched so that they appear identical to an active comparator. Positive placebo effects are common in trials of psychotropic medicines. They appear to result from the positive attribution of change to the supposed action of the tablet – a cognitive mechanism.

Psychosis: the traditional term for mental states characterized by delusions and or hallucinations. The loss of contact with reality makes patients more likely to be vulnerable or dangerous.

Randomized controlled trial: a clinical experiment in which patients are assigned at random to two or more different treatment groups; the outcomes are compared with the control group (e.g. those receiving placebo or the current 'gold standard' therapy).

Tardive dyskinesia: the abnormal involuntary movement disorder associated with long-term use of typical antipsychotics. It generally involves spontaneous movement of the lips and face, and arises after prolonged treatment (usually years).

Unipolar disorder: unipolar patients experience only one pole of mood disorder. In practice, this diagnosis can apply only to depression – major depressive disorder – because DSM-IV defines bipolar disorder with reference only to mania. Unipolar mania is, however, extremely rare.

Introduction

Bipolar disorder, or manic-depression, is a disease with a long history. In antiquity, Greek clinicians described both the euphoria and psychosis associated with manic states, and the despair and suicidal inclinations associated with melancholia, the older word for depression. However, the great distinction between 'manic-depressive insanity' and other forms of psychosis – especially dementia praecox and schizophrenia – was first made explicitly by Emil Kraepelin in the late 19th century. Like other psychiatrists at the time, his observations were confined to the clientele of asylums. Therefore, he saw the worst cases of affective disorder and its most extreme manifestations in psychotic depression or mania.

Kraepelin did not distinguish between patients with both elevation and depression of mood, and those who showed only psychotic, but unipolar, depression. The emphasis on bipolarity is modern and arose from the work of Angst and Perris in the 1960s. It is the distinction that they drew between bipolar and unipolar cases that now highlights mania and mood elevation as the defining feature of bipolar disorder.

A central feature of the Kraepelinian dichotomy between affective psychosis and schizophrenia was the difference that he discerned in

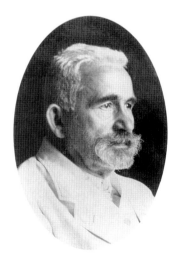

Figure 1 Emil Kraepelin (1856–1926) first made the distinction between 'manic-depressive insanity' and other forms of psychosis. Source: The Wellcome Library, London

the outcome of the two conditions. The outcome in schizophrenia he saw as being consistent: very often, it is poor with residual symptoms, cognitive impairments and social withdrawal. By contrast, manic-depression – bipolar disorder – is compatible with complete recovery. Unfortunately, however, we also know that such complete recovery is the exception rather than the rule. Outcomes, and the need to improve them, are one of the major reasons why the treatment of bipolar disorder must be moved forward.

Bipolar disorder has been a neglected disease, certainly by comparison with schizophrenia. We hope that this is changing. We now have an increased understanding of its prevalence and neurobiology, as the advances of the last two decades are applied to psychiatric disorder, and treatment has improved as researchers have explored the illness as a target for new classes of medicines. There has also been a growth in interest in formal psychological interventions for bipolar disorder which may turn out to have a major part to play in the management of an illness whose origins appear to be largely biological. In parallel with these essentially scientific advances, there has been a much greater appreciation of the plight of patients with the illness, the impact it has on their lives and the many failures, big and small, of the services provided to help them.

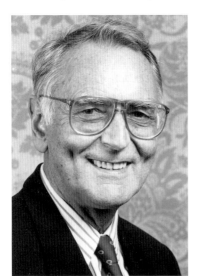

Figure 2 Jules Angst has played a major role in increasing our understanding of the diagnosis and course of bipolar disorder.

These relatively recent developments have paved the way for a much more unified view of the illness worldwide, and have facilitated clearer agreement on the vital research agenda for the next decade. The authors have had the privilege of participating in the development of this consensus and the planning for future studies.

This book provides a brief synopsis of current understanding and strategies. We hope it will be of interest to anyone whose mission is to treat bipolar patients and to champion their cause. This includes primary care physicians with an interest in the disorder, psychiatrists, therapists and nurses, all of whom can provide so much help to individual patients in their care.

Finally, we hope that patients and their families may want to use this book. They can provide the ultimate stimulus to improve practice by directly challenging their doctors to keep up-to-date and alert to new developments. We hope they will also participate enthusiastically in research into the causes and nature of bipolar disorder, and the randomized trials that can improve its treatment.

The lasting contribution of investigators in the 20th century has been to formalize the criteria by which psychiatric diagnoses are made. The *Diagnostic and Statistical Manual of Mental Disorders*, Fourth Edition (DSM-IV), which includes the latest revisions to these criteria, gives clear and explicit rules for diagnosing bipolar disorder. Such diagnoses are sometimes criticized for their lack of validity. In fact, their strength is their reliability, which allows us to be confident that when we describe bipolar disorder we are describing something that others could recognize in their own practice or experience.

Diagnosis is a fundamental activity for doctors. It implies that there has been application of a medical model. We believe that the medical model is useful in diagnosing bipolar disorder – indeed, we cannot see a viable or reliable alternative. However, by a medical model, we mean a unifying scientific discipline, not an exclusive reliance on medicines. This point is important to us and we return to it in Chapter 4.

Mania

The diagnosis of mania depends on the recognition of key symptoms (Table 1.1), which must either be present for at least 1 week or have resulted in hospital admission. Manic symptoms result in severe impairment of the normal ability to function; this is the additional criterion that defines mania in the absence of admission to hospital. Mania varies in severity from severe psychotic exhaustion on the one hand, to a mischievous state of elation accompanied by very bad judgment on the other.

Manic states must always be taken seriously because of the potential for patients to do themselves irreparable physical harm by taking risks, especially when driving, or social harm from imprudence, excessive spending or sexual indiscretions. It is therefore almost always essential to recognize the disorder and to initiate treatment as soon as possible.

Psychotic features are relatively common in mania and, according to most surveys, are seen in about 50% of cases. They usually manifest as

TABLE 1.1

DSM-IV criteria for mania (mania defines bipolar I disorder)

The core symptoms of the disease must be present for 1 week and/or require hospital admission:

1 A distinct period of abnormally and persistently elevated, expansive or irritable mood, lasting at least 1 week (or any duration, if hospitalization is necessary)

2 During the period of mood disturbance, three (or more) of the following symptoms have persisted (four if the mood is only irritable) and have been present to a significant degree:

a. inflated self-esteem or grandiosity

b. decreased need for sleep (e.g. feels rested after only 3 hours of sleep)

c. more talkative than usual or pressure to keep talking

d. flight of ideas or subjective experience that thoughts are racing

e. distractibility (i.e. attention too easily drawn to unimportant or irrelevant external stimuli)

f. increase in goal-directed activity (either socially, at work or school, or sexually) or psychomotor agitation

g. excessive involvement in pleasurable activities that have a high potential for painful consequences (e.g. engaging in unrestrained buying sprees, sexual indiscretions, or foolish business investments)

3 The symptoms do not meet criteria for a 'mixed episode'

4 The mood disturbance is sufficiently severe to cause marked impairment in occupational functioning or in usual social activities or relationships with others, or to necessitate hospitalization to prevent harm to self or others, or there are psychotic features

5 The symptoms are not due to the direct physiological effects of a substance (e.g. a drug of abuse, a medication, or other treatment) or a general medical condition (e.g. hyperthyroidism)

delusions that are mood congruent. They are often grandiose, reflecting the elevation of mood, and may, for example, over-estimate the personal qualities of the patient in regard to their attractiveness, ability and power. Some patients with mania show mood-incongruent symptoms – delusions and hallucinations very similar to those seen in schizophrenia. A full schizophrenia syndrome can coexist with mania and it is then called schizo-affective psychosis. Schizo-affective states are probably best thought of as a combination of the two recognized syndromes rather than a separate group.

Bipolar I disorder is diagnosed on the basis of mania alone in DSM-IV, although there is often a history of depression, and certainly a risk of future depression. However, the course of the illness is not individually predictable.

Hypomania

Functional impairment underpins a crucial distinction that is made in DSM-IV between mania and hypomania. Hypomania is a state that is not associated with significant functional impairment and may be viewed by patients as positively desirable. This state is arbitrarily required to last 4 days or more to meet DSM-IV diagnostic criteria.

A state of hypomania may be the prelude to mania in bipolar I disorder or it may be the greatest elevation in mood that an individual ever experiences. In the former case, it is an indication for vigilance and usually also for active treatment to avoid mania. In the latter, hypomania in a patient with major depression constitutes a diagnosis of bipolar II disorder.

The problem of how to treat bipolar II disorder is assuming increasing importance, but presently lacks almost any evidence base beyond anecdote and observation. Furthermore, hypomania is not a familiar diagnosis to many clinicians. Patients seldom *complain* of hypomania and, moreover, the term is widely misused – almost out of a sense of politeness – to describe mania. Failure to detect hypomania will, of course, render clinicians oblivious to the existence of bipolar II disorder, which will usually present as major depression.

Mixed states

The classic view of mania emphasizes euphoria, expansiveness and overactivity. There are, however, states of mania that are much more an admixture of both manic and depressive features. A particular additional risk with such illnesses is suicide, which is almost always correlated with the presence of depressive symptoms.

The recognition of mixed states may pose significant diagnostic problems even for experienced psychiatrists, because presentations are difficult to stereotype as recognizable vignettes. The two most common forms are rapidly alternating mania and depression, or a severe depression with complete absence of euphoria or humor but showing labile periods of pressured, irritable hostility and paranoia.

Major depression

The depressions associated with bipolar disorder have much in common with those experienced by patients with other types of depressive illness. The diagnostic criteria for major depression in DSM-IV require that five or more of the key symptoms are present for more than 2 weeks. As shown in Table 1.2, there are many key symptoms and therefore many ways of becoming depressed.

On average, certain features are more common in bipolar patients than in those with unipolar disorders. Marked psychomotor retardation is common, together with psychotic depression in younger people and atypical features of depression, such as hypersomnia. A first-degree relative with bipolar depression should also suggest a bipolar diagnosis in a patient with major depression.

Depression is usually the predominant abnormality of mood and an important cause of functional impairment in bipolar patients, and contributes to their increased mortality from suicide.

Minor bipolar disorder

Bipolar I and II disorders are broadly accepted categories in DSM-IV. Other, generally less severe, manifestations of mood elevation and depression are now also thought to merit recognition as bipolar disorder. These include recurrent brief depression or mania that has many or all of the features of the full syndromes, but presents for much shorter periods of time, and cyclothymia, which is mood variation that typically takes place over many years with sub-syndromal mood depression or elation as a frequent feature of an individual's personal experience. These states are of interest because they may be harbingers of the major syndromes, or they can offer clues to the etiology, especially heritability.

TABLE 1.2

DSM-IV criteria for major depression

Five (or more) of the following symptoms have been present during the same 2-week period and represent a change from previous functioning; at least one of the symptoms is either (1) depressed mood or (2) loss of interest or pleasure. Note: do not include symptoms that are clearly due to a general medical condition, or mood-incongruent delusions or hallucinations

1 Depressed mood most of the day, nearly every day, as indicated by either subjective report (e.g. feels sad or empty) or observation made by others (e.g. appears tearful). Note: in children and adolescents, can be irritable mood

2 Markedly diminished interest or pleasure in all, or almost all, activities most of the day, nearly every day (as indicated by either subjective account or observation made by others)

3 Significant weight loss when not dieting or weight gain (e.g. a change of more than 5% of body weight in a month), or decrease or increase in appetite nearly every day. In children, consider failure to make expected weight gains

4 Insomnia or hypersomnia nearly every day

5 Psychomotor agitation or retardation nearly every day (observable by others, not merely subjective feelings of restlessness or being slowed down)

6 Fatigue or loss of energy nearly every day

7 Feelings of worthlessness or excessive or inappropriate guilt (which may be delusional) nearly every day (not merely self-reproach or guilt about being sick)

8 Diminished ability to think or concentrate, or indecisiveness, nearly every day (either by subjective account or as observed by others)

9 Recurrent thoughts of death (not just fear of dying), recurrent suicidal ideation without a specific plan, or a suicide attempt or a specific plan for committing suicide

Rapid cycling

Patients with four or more episodes of mania, hypomania, mixed state or depression in the preceding 12 months are described as rapid cycling. This definition includes patients who show remission between these episodes and those who cycle continuously (or switch continually) from one polarity to the other without euthymia. The lifetime risk of rapid cycling is around 16%; however, it persists indefinitely in only a few patients.

Rapid cycling is weakly associated with female gender, bipolar II disorder, current hypothyroidism and a less robust response to lithium (especially the depressive component). It may often be difficult to treat. Rapid cycling may be preceded by exposure to antidepressants, and worsened by treatment with antidepressants, but there is no proof of a causal relationship.

Comorbidity

Patients with bipolar disorder often also meet the criteria for other psychiatric diagnoses, of which the most important are anxiety-related disorders and substance misuse. These disorders occur much more frequently than might be expected from the rates in the general population.

As many as 93% of bipolar I patients may have an anxiety disorder at some stage in their life. This is such a high figure that anxiety symptoms may be viewed as part of the bipolar phenotype. Anxiety disorders encountered in bipolar patients include, in descending order of prevalence: panic, generalized anxiety disorder and obsessive–compulsive disorder.

Anxiety symptoms or syndromes are sometimes the earliest symptoms that a patient experiences. They are clinically most salient between acute episodes and in bipolar depression, although many patients describe anxiety as a component of their manic experience as well, particularly as a prodrome. Indeed, anxiety symptoms may sometimes be the chief determinant of clinical outcome.

Substance misuse is also a common and clinically significant comorbidity of bipolar I and II disorder. It may be driven in part by the potential of addictive drugs to relieve anxiety and elevate mood. Appropriate assessment and effective treatment of significant substance or alcohol misuse is important, because it can improve compliance and bipolar outcomes.

Drug-induced psychosis

A drug-induced psychosis, as defined in DSM-IV, should either disappear with the clearance of the offending drug or be a transient phenomenon of drug withdrawal. This is quite a restrictive diagnosis. Unfortunately, the term is often used in clinical practice whenever mania is associated with the use of a variety of stimulant drugs. Where manic states are sustained, a diagnosis of 'drug-induced psychosis' is likely to be wrong, and misleading. Even if a stimulant drug appears to have acted as a trigger, the diagnosis of bipolar disorder is likely to be more appropriate.

Prescribed medications, most commonly levodopa and corticosteroids, are also associated with secondary mania. Thyroid disease, multiple sclerosis or any lesion(s) involving right-sided subcortical or cortical areas may similarly be a cause of secondary mania and should be considered in the differential diagnosis. An underlying physical diagnosis is most likely in mature patients with a late onset of mood symptoms.

Antidepressant-induced mania. Antidepressants may be a trigger for mania and hypomania. This issue will be discussed at length in the chapter covering acute treatment (Chapter 6), but it is also a problem for diagnosis. In DSM-IV, mania or hypomania induced by antidepressants is not regarded as diagnostic of bipolar disorder. The diagnosis can, of course, be made if patients have had a manic episode while off medicines – but what of patients who switch to mania or hypomania only when prescribed antidepressants? There is likely to be a revision in future DSM editions to recognize a bipolar diagnosis in these patients too, but DSM-IV currently leaves their diagnosis in limbo. The approach to their treatment should certainly follow the principles we describe for bipolar patients who do meet DSM-IV criteria.

Key points – definitions: diagnosis and comorbidity

- DSM-IV provides the preferred framework for diagnosis of bipolar disorder.
- Mania defines bipolar I disorder.
- Bipolar II disorder is defined by hypomania, which is *not* associated with significant functional impairment, together with major depression.
- Major depression is similar for the unipolar and bipolar patient, although psychosis, retardation and atypical features, or a first-degree relative with bipolar disorder, should suggest a bipolar diagnosis.
- Suicide is an important lifelong risk for bipolar patients.
- Briefer, less severe mood elevations are also described in patients with depression and are currently extending our concept of the bipolar spectrum.
- Hypomania or mania induced by antidepressants or stimulants usually implies a bipolar diagnosis.
- Anxiety disorders, and substance and alcohol misuse are the most common significant clinical comorbidities and negatively affect outcome.

Personality disorder

In DSM-IV, personality disorder may be an 'axis II' accompaniment of any 'axis I' psychiatric diagnosis. Accordingly, a diagnosis of bipolar I disorder may be made in someone also judged to have a disorder of personality. However, the behavioral disturbances of young people with manic mood elevation pose a particular challenge. If they are interpreted as personality based, not illness based, the 'personality diagnosis' may blind the clinician to bipolar disorder. The failure to diagnose bipolar disorder is a far greater disservice to the patient than to 'miss' the personality problem.

Borderline personality disorder is defined by criteria that include 'mood swings', deliberate self-harm and relationship difficulties, but requires onset of these symptoms as a constant feature before the age of 18. The possible overlap between borderline symptoms, bipolar spectrum and ultrarapid-cycling bipolar disorder remains most uncertain.

Diagnosis sets the scene for the important questions: what are these mood disorders, why do people develop abnormal mood states, and what should we try to do about it?

Key references

American Psychiatric Association. *Diagnostic and Statistical Manual for Mental Disorders (DSM-IV).* Washington, DC: American Psychiatric Association, 1994.

Cassidy F, Forest K, Murry E, Carroll BJ. A factor analysis of the signs and symptoms of mania. *Arch Gen Psychiatry* 1998;55(1):27–32.

Goodwin GM. Hypomania – what's in a name? *Br J Psychiatry* 2002;180: 94–5.

Kendell RE. Diagnosis and classification of functional psychoses. *Br Med Bull* 1987;43(3):499–513.

Mitchell PB, Wilhelm K, Parker G et al. The clinical features of bipolar depression: a comparison with matched major depressive disorder patients. *J Clin Psychiatry* 2001;62(3):212–16.

Salloum IM, Thase ME. Impact of substance abuse on the course and treatment of bipolar disorder. *Bipolar Disord* 2000;2(3 Pt 2):269–80.

Genetics

After establishing their name, it is said that the second question asked of all new patients seen at the Maudsley Hospital (London, UK) in the last 60 years has been "Are you a twin?". If you are a twin with any illness, then whether or not your brother or sister is also affected provides vital information about whether or not the condition is inherited. Identical twins share 100% of their genes, while non-identical twins share 50%. There is therefore a higher risk of any inherited illness or trait also being expressed in the co-twin if they are a monozygotic pair rather than a dizygotic pair. In the case of severe bipolar I disorder, the risk has been estimated to be as high as 80%; in other words, the disorder is highly heritable.

Bipolar disorder will therefore run in families. Furthermore, diagnoses that are related, in a genetic sense, to bipolar disorder may also appear in families at an increased rate. When the rates of illnesses in first-degree relatives of index cases are studied, it is found that the risk of bipolar disorder in the families of bipolar patients is about 6%, compared with a rate of around 0.5% in the general population. The risk of psychosis (usually schizophrenia) is similarly increased in the relatives of patients with schizophrenia (Figure 2.1). Figure 2.1 also shows the unexpected finding that, in the families of index cases with schizophrenia, bipolar or unipolar disorder, the risk of unipolar depression is increased approximately equally. In addition, there may be some increase in the risk of psychosis in patients with bipolar disorder.

If we think of these different diagnoses as being largely correlated with individual genes or groups of genes, it seems that the phenotype of bipolar disorder is associated not just with 'bipolar genes', but also with genes for unipolar depression (common in relatives) and genes for psychosis (with psychotic phenotypes being encountered in relatives at a much lower frequency). Index cases with schizo-affective disorder have an excess of both bipolar disorder and psychosis among their relatives (not shown in Figure 2.1), which is what would be predicted

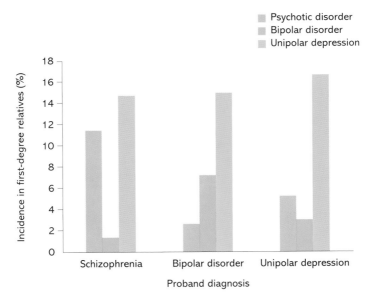

Psychotic disorder
Bipolar disorder
Unipolar depression

Figure 2.1 Incidence of different diagnoses in the families of patients with different index illnesses. A patient with schizophrenia will have more family members with psychosis than bipolar disorder, and the converse is the case for a patient with bipolar disorder. Notice the increased risk of major depression in the families of patients with schizophrenia, bipolar disorder and unipolar depression. Modified from Gershon ES et al. *Arch Gen Psychiatry* 1982:39(10):1157–67.

if such cases have the genes predisposing to both disorders.

This suggests that bipolar disorder is a complex phenotype, with inheritance likely to be determined by a number of functionally related genes, as illustrated schematically in Figure 2.2. This has turned out to be the case in most relatively common physical diseases. It is still possible that unusually informative families exist with simpler inheritance – and clearer clues to the fundamental neurobiology – but, if so, they remain to be discovered. We should not expect, and we do not find, clear evidence for single-gene inheritance or genome scans suggesting single loci homogeneously related to bipolar disorder in reasonable sized samples.

Instead, the hunt is for genes of relatively modest effect, some of which may contribute to a risk for depression, others of which may

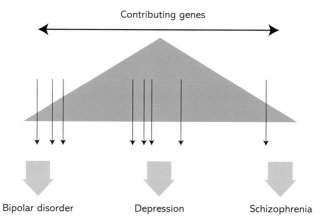

Figure 2.2 Illustration of the polygenic inheritance of bipolar disorder. The red triangle represents a spectrum of *functionally* related genes which together may contribute to a range of psychiatric disorders (shown as green arrows). The vertical lines represent polymorphic genes that may actually act in a single individual to produce bipolar disorder. The numbers of genes that make up the relevant genes and the actual numbers required for illness to arise are unknown, but may be large.

contribute specifically to a risk for mania or psychosis. A mix of genetic factors seems necessary to explain why the phenotypes of mania, depression and schizophrenia show the variation that they do. The challenge will be to tease out the function of individual genes or groups of genes acting in development or in relevant neuronal systems.

The issue of heritability is not just an issue for clinical scientists. It matters a great deal to patients with bipolar disorder and their families. In the most common case, in which the spouse of the person with bipolar disorder has no history of mood disorder, the risk of their child being affected is of the order of 6%. This can be expressed in a frightening way as representing a 12-fold increase in risk over the general population rate of 0.5% or, less alarmingly, as a 1 in 17 chance that the child will have bipolar disorder. Both expressions of risk are correct, but the latter is probably what matters most for the patient and family. Of course, other unions may give rise to higher risks, especially if both parents have mood disorder or come from families in which severe mood disorder is prominent.

Neurobiology

To say that bipolar disorder is largely determined by genes is currently a true, but trite, statement. It is known that genes code for proteins and that proteins make up the enzymes, receptors and intracellular signals released by receptor activation (second messengers), on which neurotransmitters act in the brain. Genes also control the growth and development of neurons. There are, therefore, a myriad of ways in which genetic variation could have an impact on a mature nervous system.

In the case of bipolar disorder, and unlike schizophrenia, there is little evidence for an environmental trigger factor or a neurodevelopmental defect. Most children who will develop bipolar disorder appear to reach adulthood without showing obvious developmental, behavioral or temperamental abnormalities. It is, however, too early to say that there will be no important, measurable, behavioral variations associated with bipolar disorder, because it is currently an area of active investigation (see below).

It is commonly supposed that most severe mental illnesses have a trigger. Most cases of depression, for example, are preceded by life events. This is also true, to a lesser extent, of the first onset of schizophrenic psychoses. While less studied, the onset of mania may also be weakly associated with a life event or events, although not clearly 'negative' ones. However, because life events are common in young people and bipolar disorder starts at a young age, the specificity of this relationship is difficult to establish. A trigger may sometimes be necessary, but it is never sufficient to cause mania. Triggers have the same relationship to the real causes of severe bipolar disorder as a spark has to gunpowder. The persistent finding of hypothalamic–pituitary–adrenal (HPA) axis dysfunction in mood disorder (see page 26) may eventually explain how 'social' stressors can be represented as *physiological* constructs.

How acute states of mood disturbance develop on a background of euthymia remains uncertain. There have been many studies describing biological abnormalities in depression, and to a lesser extent in mania, but the findings barely add up to a coherent theory. Acute states of mania and depression produce such profound disturbances of

23

physiology and behavior that it should, perhaps, come as no surprise that many systems are found to be perturbed in some way. Unfortunately, such changes may be epiphenomena. It is much more interesting when any biological abnormality is found that characterizes the euthymic condition and gives a basis for understanding the vulnerability to relapse that typifies the disorder.

Psychopharmacology

Greater understanding of the neurobiology of manic or depressive states would provide candidate systems in which to look for the predicted genetic effects. The greatest clues to the etiology have come from the toxic effects of stimulants and the fortuitous discovery of medicines that seem to be effective.

Mania. There are many similarities between manic states and the changes that take place in volunteers given euphoriant doses of amphetamine. In both cases, there is an elevation in mood and energy, together with a reduced need for sleep. It is curious, therefore, that the 'dopamine hypothesis' is usually associated with schizophrenia, depending as it does on the less common *psychotomimetic* effects of amphetamine. Amphetamine provokes a state corresponding to mania more reliably than to schizophrenia. This places excess release of monoamines, especially dopamine, as a central mechanism that possibly underlies the psychopathology of mania. The findings of studies on transmitter metabolites in cerebrospinal fluid, which were conducted in the 1970–80s, support the idea of increased neurotransmitter turnover in mania.

The central role of dopamine overactivity in mania is supported by the now very convincing evidence that atypical antipsychotics, all of which occupy the dopamine D2 receptor, are effective antimanic agents (see Chapter 6). In addition, depletion of the substrates for dopamine synthesis (the amino acids tyrosine and phenylalanine) attenuates the effects of amphetamine in animals and man, and is also antimanic. Some aspects of the cognitive performance of manic subjects, such as increased distractibility on performing tasks requiring attention, may also be related to excess dopamine function. The relevant neuroanatomy lies in the connections that exist between the striatum and the frontal cortex, and possibly the direct projections of dopamine neurons to the frontal cortex (Figure 2.3).

Dopamine may not, however, offer a complete explanation for mania. Mania is also treated with lithium and relapse may be reliably triggered by lithium withdrawal. The pharmacology of lithium only indirectly influences dopamine function.

Depression. Contemporary ideas about depression have been strongly influenced by our understanding of serotonergic function in the brain. When the availability of the serotonin substrate, tryptophan, is depleted by loading with other amino acids, recovered individuals with recurrent unipolar depression show a return of depressive symptoms. Such observations suggest a very strong and direct link between serotonin function in the brain and the risk of depression in vulnerable subjects. However, efforts to demonstrate symptom return after depletion of tryptophan in bipolar I patients have failed. It therefore remains

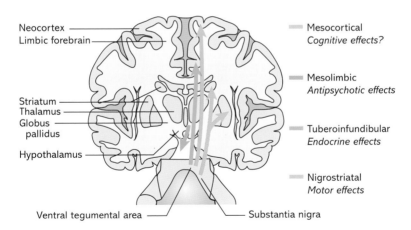

Figure 2.3 The connections that exist between the striatum and the frontal cortex, and possibly the direct projections of the dopamine neurons to the frontal cortex, may be relevant to the role of dopamine in attention and reward. The globus pallidus is concerned with motor activity, and the projections to the pituitary exert inhibitory control over the release of prolactin.

uncertain whether serotonin plays a fundamental role in the biology of bipolar depression as it appears to do in unipolar cases. It could, and probably does, still provide a pathway for treatment, because selective serotonin reuptake inhibitors appear to be effective in bipolar depression.

Norepinephrine (noradrenaline) rivals serotonin for the attention of neuroscientists interested in depression. Its depletion may also result in depression under some circumstances. Patients who have recovered from acute episodes of mania or depression show a pattern of cognitive impairment that is compatible with a noradrenergic deficit. It is possible that some noradrenergic projections are impaired by repeated episodes of illness, resulting in an increased risk of depression and an enduring deficit of sustained attention.

Endocrine function

There is a persistent, but not entirely consistent, theme of disturbed endocrine function in mood disorder, including bipolar disorder. A raised cortisol output is observed in severe depression and mania, but tends to normalize on recovery. The meaning of this phenomenon is still uncertain. The HPA axis can be tested by observing endogenous cortisol secretion after administration of the exogenous glucocorticoid, dexamethasone (the dexamethasone suppression test or DST). Suppression occurs when inhibitory feedback to the hypothalamus is mediated by the glucocorticoid receptor; non-suppression of endogenous cortisol occurs in abnormal states, such as Cushing's disease. Non-suppression of cortisol implies either reduced feedback and/or enhanced central drive for its release. The DST was shown to have a high specificity and sensitivity for severe depression compared with controls in early studies, but is less discriminating when comparing different patient groups. There appears to be hypertrophy of the adrenal glands in major depression, with a measurable increase in size on magnetic resonance imaging (MRI), and an enhanced response to a given dose of corticotropin. Like the hypercortisolemia, the MRI change is reversible on recovery. However, relatively impaired glucocorticoid feedback has also been described in those relatives of depressed patients who do not have mood disorder and in euthymic bipolar patients.

It is unclear whether endogenous cortisol actually contributes to the clinical picture of depression and mania by a direct action on the brain; if so, it may mediate at least part of the postulated stress/diathesis in mood disorder. Exogenous cortisol administration is certainly associated with affective symptoms. Acute dosing can precipitate euphoria and, in bipolar I patients, the full syndrome of mania. Chronic treatment or excessive long-term cortisol secretion can produce depressive symptoms, as in Cushing's disease. If 'cortisol toxicity' does indeed contribute to mood disorders, antagonism of cortisol's action could have important psychotropic effects. Convincing evidence is awaited.

Although steroids are measured in the extracellular compartment, the primary actions are currently understood to be on intracellular receptors. It is striking that the hypercortisolemia of mood disorder is not associated with the metabolic changes seen in Cushing's disease. This is puzzling unless it is hypothesized that transport of steroids across the plasma membrane may be disturbed in mood disorder. From this hypothesis follows an interesting new idea that high extracellular levels of cortisol could coexist or even be provoked by low local levels of intracellular cortisol.

Other endocrine abnormalities

Hyperthyroidism is characterized by increased anxiety and emotional lability; it may even present as hypomania or mania. Hypothyroidism is classically associated with a reversible dementia, although depressive features may also be prominent. As thyroid dysfunction commonly disrupts the psyche, does psychiatric disorder have reciprocal associations with thyroid dysfunction? Abnormalities of the thyroid axis in bipolar disorder have often been described. Unfortunately, there is a particular confounding factor – the use of lithium. Lithium interferes with the peripheral action of thyrotropin in the thyroid, and tends to raise thyrotropin and lower thyroid hormone levels. Nevertheless, mild hypothyroidism appears to be associated with rapid cycling and the thyrotropin response to thyrotropin-releasing hormone is blunted in some patients with depression. Furthermore, thyroid hormones have been used in the treatment of rapid cycling and refractory depression. There is also evidence that thyroxine has important interactions with neurotransmitter systems within the brain; if these are abnormally regulated in mood disorder – norepinephrine may be a particular candidate – then the basis for these often neglected clinical associations might prove extremely interesting.

Biological rhythms and sleep disturbance

The seasonality and cyclicity of bipolar disorder suggests that the sleep–wake cycle may play a fundamental role in the pathophysiology. Patients with severe depression may respond to sleep deprivation with a transient increase in mood. Sleep disturbance is associated with and may contribute to processes that initiate the onset of mania. It remains a reasonable hypothesis that sleep disturbance is a final common pathway through which a variety of stressors may operate to trigger mood episodes in patients with bipolar I disorder.

Functional neuropathology

Classically, brain diseases have a neuropathology that is often characterized by the appearance of abnormal proteins. These can provide the first molecular signature of the disorder, like the plaques and tangles in Alzheimer's disease. Psychiatric disorders do not generally have a pathology that is detectable on gross inspection or under light microscopy. This has led to the designation of psychiatric disorder, perhaps tastelessly, as a graveyard for pathologists. Some objections to a medical approach to psychiatry also rest on this apparent failure.

In recent years, improved methods for quantifying cell number and synaptic connectivity have led to the discovery that certain areas of the limbic cortex are, after all, abnormal in patients with mood disorder. The changes in cell number now detectable with improved counting methodology appear to be most striking in the glial cell population, but the associated changes in synaptic density obviously involve neurons. Although the abnormality is quantitative rather than qualitative, it could constitute the basis for the subtle but pervasive symptoms of mood disorder, and explain the tendency for recurrence. Caution is still in order, because there may be alternative explanations. However, a

functional or even synaptic neuropathology is a plausible unifying
explanation for much of what is seen clinically.

Neuroimaging

At present, neuroimaging has revealed nothing that is helpful for the
diagnosis, management and treatment of bipolar disorder. However, as
techniques are refined, imaging is likely to contribute much more to our

---

Key points – etiology

- Bipolar I disorder, especially identified as hospitalized mania, is
  a highly heritable condition. The present evidence suggests a
  contribution from multiple genes of modest or small effect.
- Unlike schizophrenia, there is little evidence for an
  environmental factor or a neurodevelopmental defect.
- Family studies show an excess of unipolar depression and
  psychosis among bipolar patients, suggesting that the polygenic
  inheritance is expressed as a variety of related phenotypes.
- Dopamine hyperactivity appears directly implicated in the
  neurobiology of manic symptoms.
- Bipolar depression, unlike unipolar forms, may not be securely
  linked to decreased function of serotonin. Norepinephrine
  may be implicated in bipolar depression and there may be
  enduring deficits in sustained attention in euthymic bipolar
  patients.
- Cortisol and thyroid hormones have been implicated in mood
  disorder. An acute excess of either tends to produce euphoria.
  Long-term hypercortisolemia may produce depression.
  Abnormalities of the hypothalamic–pituitary–adrenal and
  thyroid axes are often described in euthymic bipolar
  patients.
- Sleep is similarly disrupted in mania and depression. A direct
  euphoriant effect of sleep deprivation may be relevant to the
  evolution of the manic state.

---

understanding of abnormal structure and connectivity in the brains of patients with bipolar disorder. The key hypothesis is that neural networks regulating emotional processing in the brain are somehow vulnerable to acute decompensation – the episodes we see as clinicians. This vulnerability is very likely to be expressed in abnormal connectivity, which is potentially detectable in life with sensitive methods such as diffusion tensor imaging, positron emission tomography or spectroscopy. Moreover, repeated episodes of illness may themselves cause additional damage to these networks and make their further disruption more detectable by imaging methods. Today, the prospects for real conceptual and practical advances are more exciting than they have been for many years.

Key references

Clark L, Iversen SD, Goodwin GM. Sustained attention deficit in bipolar disorder. *Br J Psychiatry* 2002;180:313–9.

Cummings JL, Mendez MF. Secondary mania with focal cerebrovascular lesions. *Am J Psychiatry* 1984;141(9):1084–7.

Drevets WC. Prefrontal cortical-amygdalar metabolism in major depression. *Ann NY Acad Sci* 1999;877:614–37.

Gershon ES, Hamovit J, Guroff JJ et al. A family study of schizoaffective, bipolar I, bipolar II, unipolar, and normal control probands. *Arch Gen Psychiatry* 1982;39(10):1157–67.

Goodwin FK, Jamison KR. *Bipolar Disorder.* Oxford: Oxford University Press, 1990.

Harrison PJ. The neuropathology of primary mood disorder. *Brain* 2002;125(Pt 7):1428–49.

McTavish SF, McPherson MH, Harmer CJ et al. Antidopaminergic effects of dietary tyrosine depletion in healthy subjects and patients with manic illness. *Br J Psychiatry* 2001;179:356–60.

Nestler EJ, Gould E, Manji H. Preclinical models: status of basic research in depression. *Biol Psychiatry* 2002;52(6):503–28.

Potash JB, DePaulo J-R Jr. Searching high and low: a review of the genetics of bipolar disorder. *Bipolar Disord* 2000;2(1):8–26.

Smith KA, Fairburn CG, Cowen PJ. Relapse of depression after rapid depletion of tryptophan. *Lancet* 1997;349(9056):915–19.

Videbech P. MRI findings in patients with affective disorder: a meta-analysis. *Acta Psychiatr Scand* 1997;96(3):157–68.

Wehr TA, Sack DA, Rosenthal NE. Sleep reduction as a final common pathway in the genesis of mania. *Am J Psychiatry* 1987;144(2):201–4.

Bipolar I disorder, defined by the occurrence of mania and usually by hospital admission, is a relatively rare condition with a lifetime incidence of approximately 0.5% in the general population. The lifetime incidence of bipolar II disorder diagnosed using DSM-IV criteria is also probably less than 1%. Again using DSM-IV criteria, unipolar depression is by far the commonest mood disorder in the community – 21% of the Zurich sample shown on the left-hand side of Figure 3.1.

The diagnosis of bipolar II disorder remains controversial because of the boundary of hypomania with normality, rather than its boundary with mania. The issue is deceptively simple: how to draw the line between a patient who has experienced episodes of elation and one who has not. It turns out that many people experience and describe short-term changes in mood that fail to meet the DSM-IV criteria for hypomania. However, the phenomenon is often associated with other morbidity (e.g. depression, deliberate self-harm and substance misuse) and, on this basis, Angst has argued for a more liberal definition of hypomania. The more liberal the definition, the more inclusive it becomes, bringing cases of major depression into what is often called the 'bipolar spectrum'. The effect of this expansion of the concept of hypomania is an inflation of the bipolar diagnosis shown in Figure 3.1.

The clinical message, already emphasized in Chapter 1, is a relatively straightforward one. In addition to diagnosing depression in patients presenting to primary care physicians or indeed to psychiatrists, inquiries should also be made about periods of excessive energy, decreased need for sleep, heightened sexual interest, increased risk taking, enhanced cognitive ability, or elation. At present, a positive response to such inquiries and a provisional diagnosis of bipolar spectrum disorder is not a clear indication for action. It is, however, an indication for caution, particularly in the use of antidepressants (see below).

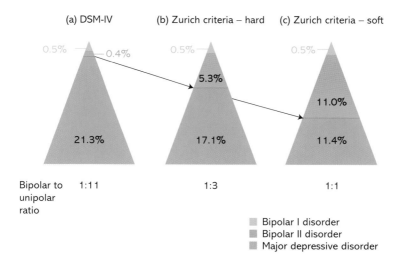

(a) DSM-IV   (b) Zurich criteria – hard   (c) Zurich criteria – soft

Bipolar I disorder
Bipolar II disorder
Major depressive disorder

Figure 3.1 The lifetime incidence of bipolar disorder depends on how bipolar II disorder is defined. (a) Applying DSM-IV criteria, the lifetime incidence of bipolar I and II disorder together is about 1%. Unipolar major depressive disorder is much more common under this definition. If the diagnosis of bipolar II disorder is liberalized, the number of patients with major depressive disorder who are re-classified as having bipolar II disorder will expand. (b) and (c) Expansion of the percentage of bipolar II patients for successively more inclusive definitions using the Zurich criteria. The hard criteria imply behavioral consequences of hypomanic mood disturbance, while the soft criteria do not. Data and Zurich criteria from Angst J et al. (2003).

Burden of disease

Mood disorders are among the leading cause of morbidity and mortality in Western and emerging countries. Bipolar cases contribute disproportionately to this toll. Morbidity is particularly high because the age of onset is usually young. How young remains controversial and merits a full discussion.

Children and young adults

The incidence of bipolar disorder is a function of age. Although a first episode of mania may be seen in patients over 80, the peak decade is

15–25 years. Anyone who has spent up to 6 months working in an acute psychiatric unit will have seen a young person admitted to hospital in a wildly excited manic state, much to the consternation of friends and family. This is the traditional view of how bipolar disorder starts.

There is now an alternative view that much earlier diagnosis should be possible if more sensitive instruments are employed. This perspective largely grows out of the experience of child and adolescent psychiatrists in the USA. The diagnosis of bipolar disorder in quite young children is becoming increasingly common. It represents another of the ways in which practice in North America is different from that in most other parts of the world, since a parallel trend has not yet been described in other countries, where bipolar disorder is almost never diagnosed before the age of 10 years.

There are at least two different ways to interpret this difference. First, there may indeed be developmental abnormalities in children who are later diagnosed as having bipolar disorder and these may be expressed as identifiable mood-congruent behavioral changes. With careful rating and attention to clinical detail, the diagnosis is now being claimed in children as young as 5 years. However, the instruments on which these claims rely are essentially modifications of adult rating scales to reflect what are interpreted as 'manic' features in children. There is an explicit softening of the edges of diagnostic criteria in an effort to detect a juvenile equivalent of the signal psychopathology seen in bipolar adults. Whether this is a valid procedure can be determined only on the basis of its predictive power: how many children detected in this way actually develop conventionally defined bipolar disorder and, just as importantly, how many do not. It is still possible for the sceptic to say that this is diagnosis inflation; the more pessimistic would argue that it may be leading to the misdiagnosis (and mistreatment) of more children than it actually satisfactorily identifies.

The second approach is to take the data at face value and propose that something is happening in the USA to make bipolar symptoms more common in children. One possible explanation is the widespread use of stimulants for the treatment of hyperactivity. Figures vary, but as many as 10% of some school populations receive stimulants for this indication and, since hyperactivity could be a precursor of bipolar disorder, it is possible that exposure to amphetamine-like agents may precipitate earlier appearance of bipolar disorder than would otherwise have occurred. There are some data from US clinics to support this. Other possibilities include nutritional and cultural factors, which may accelerate the trend of earlier expression of mood disorder in the life cycle.

For the moment, clinicians are caught between a rock and a hard place. Parents may be keen that their children should be diagnosed with bipolar disorder early so that they can receive effective treatment. However, as we attempt to diagnose positively on the basis of predictive psychopathology, we will be less reliable and more prone to initiate treatment inappropriately. The diagnosis of bipolar I disorder requires an episode meeting the full criteria for mania. This is seldom subtle and can often be reliably established during adolescence. But, in an attempt to understand the disorder, parents and family members may look back to earlier problems, presume they were part and parcel of the illness, and complain that the diagnosis was missed. Such nonspecific

Key points – epidemiology

- The lifetime incidence of bipolar I disorder is approximately 0.5%. The lifetime incidence of conservatively defined DSM-IV bipolar II disorder is also less than 1%.
- A more liberal diagnosis of hypomania will lead to a higher incidence of bipolar disorder which will include many cases now diagnosed as 'unipolar' major depression.
- Clinicians should inquire about a personal and family history of mood elevation when making a diagnosis of depression.
- Even when conservatively defined, bipolar disorder imposes a major worldwide burden of disease.
- The diagnosis of bipolar disorder in children is controversial. The incidence described in North America is much higher than in the rest of the world, where it is almost never diagnosed before the age of 10 years.

difficulties should not be indiscriminately linked with the specific development of bipolar disorder, because to do so places a burden on clinicians that even those using the most rigorous research techniques would be ill-equipped to bear.

It will be clear that this review comes at a watershed for early diagnosis. Clinicians and patients must remain on the alert for the definitive results that are expected to emerge in the next few years.

Key references

Akiskal HS, Bourgeois ML, Angst J et al. Re-evaluating the prevalence of and diagnostic composition within the broad clinical spectrum of bipolar disorders. *J Affect Disord* 2000;59 Suppl 1:S5–30.

Angst J. The emerging epidemiology of hypomania and bipolar II disorder. *J Affect Disord* 1998;50(2–3): 143–51.

Angst J, Gamma A, Benazzi F et al. Toward a re-definition of subthreshold bipolarity: epidemiology and proposed criteria for bipolar-II, minor bipolar disorders and hypomania. *J Affect Disord* 2003;73(1–2):133–46.

Harrington R, Myatt T. Is preadolescent mania the same condition as adult mania? A British perspective. *Biol Psychiatr* 2003; 53:961–9.

Harris EC, Barraclough B. Suicide as an outcome for mental disorders. A meta-analysis. *Br J Psychiatry* 1997;170:205–28.

Judd LL, Akiskal HS, Schettler PJ et al. The long-term natural history of the weekly symptomatic status of bipolar I disorder. *Arch Gen Psychiatry* 2002;59(6):530–7.

Kessler RC, Rubinow DR, Holmes C et al. The epidemiology of DSM-III-R bipolar I disorder in a general population survey. *Psychol Med* 1997;27(5):1079–89.

Murray CJL, Lopez AD. Alternative projections of mortality and disability by cause 1990–2020: Global Burden of Disease Study. *Lancet* 1997a;349:1498–1504.

Murray CJL, Lopez AD. Global mortality, disability, and the contribution of risk factors: Global Burden of Disease Study. *Lancet* 1997b;349:1436–42.

ten Have M, Vollebergh W, Bijl R, Nolen WA. Bipolar disorder in the general population in the Netherlands (prevalence, consequences and care utilisation): results from the Netherlands Mental Health Survey and Incidence Study (NEMESIS). *J Affect Disord* 2002;68(2–3):203–13.

4 The patient's perspective

It is a consistent and distressing observation, frequently made by patients with mood disorder, that their problems and suffering are not taken seriously. This is not just a failing of doctors – it extends to most people they encounter.

Depression in a variety of forms, from the mild and nagging dysphoria that may last for months to the paralysing grips of suicidal despair, is a condition that few who have not suffered it can truly claim to understand. Reality seems different after such experiences. By contrast, the euphoria and excitement of mania, the seemingly endless possibilities, the blinding insights, and the excitement of feeling powerful, active and hypersexual are experiences that may be highly valued and difficult to relinquish.

The facts given in the preceding chapters largely omit such rich personal experience in favor of a starvation diet of symptoms, diagnoses and frequencies of occurrence. On the face of it, this approach looks like a further denial of the patient's reality. It is necessary to understand that it is something different and vitally important.

Scientific psychiatry

The problem is not that clinicians wish to diminish the value of individual experience, or that they necessarily fail to understand and sympathize (although this may happen, of course). Excellent clinicians seek what is common in form or content in the stories patients tell them, not what is unique. There is a very good reason for this scientific approach to psychiatric disorders: it offers reliable knowledge, not anecdote. Indeed, all that science is, ultimately, is reliable knowledge. And it is often just such knowledge that patients seek from their doctors about their illness – how long it will last, whether it will recur, whether it runs in families and what the best treatment is.

Doctors may be wise to make neither friends of their patients, nor patients of their friends. This traditional slogan of safe practice places the science of medicine on a different basis from the content of everyday human contact.

Scientific knowledge is reliable because it is spare and reductionist. Mania is defined by reference to a checklist of symptoms – we then know what anyone using the term in a technical way actually means. It is also possible to estimate the probability of mania developing in a lifetime, and the prevalence in a population and in a service. We can then start to generate hypotheses about the underlying cause (e.g. whether or not it is genetic) and conduct trials that measure outcomes with different treatments. Investigators tend to prefer outcomes that are also clearly defined and narrow – seeming to leave out what 'matters most' to an individual in favor of what we think captures measurable, but meaningful, change in the clinical state. This approach is underpinned by the principle that if an approach is wrong, then it will be found out by our inability to replicate results and failure to move on to more fruitful hypotheses. Scientific ideas are falsifiable; anecdote and personal experience are not, and have to be judged by other quasi-literary standards.

Reliable knowledge about any natural phenomenon increases as more effort is put into research. Over the last century, medicine has generally been transformed by just such a scientific approach to the definition of illness, investigation and treatment in every specialty. In the past, every severe illness was a mysterious personal journey to death or disability to which almost any mythology could be attached. Arguably, psychiatry has been the slowest specialty to adopt science wholeheartedly and it also happens to deal with the subtlest disturbances of personal function – in emotion, thinking and behavior. However, psychiatric illnesses kill millions of people every year through suicide, and rank as leading causes of disability worldwide. If such disorders could be better treated, fewer people would die unnecessarily. That, in essence, is why doctors such as ourselves hold the views that we do and try to make our practice more scientific.

Science also provides the basis for what we want all patients to know about their illness. That knowledge may be crucial to their self-management and to the effective contribution of family and friends. It not only includes the effective use of medicines and the need for adherence to what is prescribed, though that is very important, but also includes understanding why lifestyle changes may be necessary and how specific psychological treatments may provide benefit. These are key factors in enhancement of care.

Patients' experiences

A scientific acceptance of the facts of bipolar disorder, and how to treat it, is no real barrier to listening to the stories of bipolar patients, because they are often so interesting. Indeed, there appears to be a fundamental connection between mood disorder and artistic or literary creativity. Kay Jamison's masterly survey 'Touched with Fire' makes an overwhelming case. Some of the greatest artists who have ever lived provide a treasure trove of their experience of mood disorder. The following descriptions give a brief impression of what the experience may be like.

Of mania, Kay Jamison wrote in *An Unquiet Mind*:

> *'Even now I can see in my mind's rather peculiar eye an extraordinary shattering and shifting of light; inconstant but ravishing colours laid out across miles of circling rings; and the almost imperceptible, somehow surprisingly pallid moons of this Catherine wheel of a planet. I remember singing 'Fly me to the moons' as I swept past those of Saturn ... Long after my psychosis cleared ... it became part of what one remembers forever'.[1]*

However, mania is a transient state; more stable hyperthymic traits are associated with bipolar disorder. Nigel Nicholson described Virginia Woolf's conversation thus:

> *'One would hand her a bit of information, as dull as a lump of lead, and she would hand it back glittering with diamonds. I always felt on leaving that I had drunk two glasses of excellent champagne. Virginia was a life enhancer.'[2]*

Hyperthymia and even hypomania probably provide the key to the high achievement of creative people with bipolar disorder.

The famous writers, poets, composers and artists listed in Table 4.1 almost certainly experienced severe mood disorder. Depression is the

---

[1]Cited with permission from Jamison KR. *An Unquiet Mind. A Memoir of Moods and Madness*. London: Picador, 1996.

[2]Cited with permission from Caramagno T. *The Flight of the Mind*. Berkeley: University of California Press, 1992/The Regents of the University of California.

TABLE 4.1

Famous creative artists who almost certainly experienced severe mood disorder

Writers
- Hans Christian Andersen
- Honoré de Balzac
- Samuel Clemens (Mark Twain)
- Joseph Conrad (SA)
- Charles Dickens
- Ralph Waldo Emerson
- William Faulkner (H)
- F Scott Fitzgerald (H)
- Lewis Grassic Gibbon (SA)
- Maxim Gorky (SA)
- Kenneth Graham
- Graham Greene
- Ernest Hemingway (H, S)
- Hermann Hesse (H, SA)
- Henrik Ibsen
- Henry James
- Charles Lamb (H)
- Malcolm Lowry (H, S)
- Herman Melville
- Eugene O'Neill (H, SA)
- John Ruskin (H)
- Mary Shelley
- Robert Louis Stevenson
- August Strindberg
- Leo Tolstoy
- Ivan Turgenev
- Tennessee Williams (H)
- Mary Wollstonecraft (SA)
- Virginia Woolf (H, S)

Poets
- Antonin Artaud (H)
- Charles Baudelaire (SA)
- Thomas Lovell Beddoes (S)
- John Berryman (H, S)
- William Blake
- Robert Burns
- George Gordon, Lord Byron
- Thomas Chatterton (S)
- John Clare (H)
- Samuel Taylor Coleridge
- William Cowper (H, SA)
- Hart Crane (S)
- John Davidson (S)
- Emily Dickinson
- TS Eliot (H)
- Sergei Esenin (S)
- Robert Fergusson (H)
- Oliver Goldsmith
- Thomas Gray
- Friedrich Hölderlin (H)
- Gerard Manley Hopkins
- Victor Hugo
- Randal Jarrell (H, S)
- Samuel Johnson
- John Keats
- Heinrich Von Kleist (S)
- Vachel Lindsay (S)
- Robert Lowell (H)
- Hugh MacDiarmid (H)
- Louis MacNeice
- Osip Mandelstam (H, SA)
- Vladimir Mayakovsky (S)
- Gerard de Nerval (H, S)
- Boris Pasternak (H)

- Cesare Pavese (S)
- Sylvia Plath (H, S)
- Edgar Allan Poe (SA)
- Ezra Pound (H)
- Alexander Pushkin
- Laura Riding (SA)
- Theodore Roethke (H)
- Delmore Schwartz (H)
- Anne Sexton (H, S)
- Percy Bysshe Shelley (SA)
- Torquato Tasso (H)
- Alfred, Lord Tennyson
- Dylan Thomas
- George Trakl (H, S)
- Marina Tsvetayeva (S)
- Walt Whitman

Composers

- Hector Berlioz (SA)
- Anton Bruckner (H)
- Jeremiah Clarke (S)
- John Dowland
- Edward Elgar
- Mikhail Glinka
- George Frederic Handel
- Gustav Holst
- Charles Ives
- Otto Klemperer (H)
- Orlando de Lassus
- Gustav Mahler
- Modest Mussorgsky
- Sergey Rachmaninoff
- Giocchino Rossini
- Robert Schumann (H, S)

- Alexander Scriabin
- Peter Tchaikovsky
- Peter Warlock (S)
- Hugo Wolf (H, SA)
- Bernd Alois Zimmerman (S)

Artists

- Ralph Barton (S)
- Francesco Bassano (S)
- Francesco Borromini (S)
- Richard Dadd (H)
- Edward Dayes (S)
- Paul Gauguin (SA)
- Théodore Géricault
- Hugo van der Goes
- Vincent van Gogh (H, S)
- Arshile Gorky (S)
- Philip Guston (H)
- Benjamin Haydon (S)
- Ernst Josephson (H)
- George Innes (SA)
- Ernst Ludwig Kirchner (H, S)
- Edwin Landseer (H)
- Edward Lear
- Michelangelo Buonarroti
- Edvard Munch (H)
- Jules Pascin (S)
- Georgia O'Keeffe (H)
- Jackson Pollock (H)
- Dante Gabriel Rossetti (SA)
- Mark Rothko (S)
- Nicolas de Staël (S)
- Henry Tilson (S)
- Sir David Wilkie

H, admitted at least once to an asylum or psychiatric hospital; S, suicide; SA, suicide attempt

Adapted with the permission of The Free Press, a Division of Simon & Schuster Adult Publishing Group, from *Touched with Fire: Manic-Depressive Illness and the Artistic Temperament* by Kay Redfield Jamison. © 1993 by Kay Redfield Jamison.

most pervasive consequence of bipolar disorder, and the best documented clinical state in these individuals. However, many clearly experienced mania, and showed bursts of productivity likely related to hypomania.

As we have already seen, alcohol and drug misuse are common comorbidities of bipolar disorder, and personal difficulties of all sorts may be aggravated by abnormal moods. Accordingly, many of those listed in Table 4.1 are better known for substance misuse and/or the chaos of their private lives than for the mood disorder that will often have played a causal part.

In less articulate forms, such material is also present in every outpatient clinic in which individuals with bipolar disorder are seen and, more importantly, heard.

That some of the very best poetry, literature and visual art is wrought by writers and artists from the experience of mood disorder is extraordinary. Why then is the salience in artists' lives of such illnesses itself so poorly appreciated by the general and even the literary public? There are at least two important explanations.

First, the extremes of experience that torture artists in the psychotic extremes of mania or depression do not usually provide the literal fabric for their work, however much it may indirectly inform it. Indeed, there is an exceedingly important distinction between madness and creativity. The creative thrust of psychosis tends, like that of drug intoxication, to be hollow and pointless unless there is a euthymic censor to create the work of art – creativity needs control, restraint, editorial structure. A writer's illness may be very effectively edited from their work, unless one is sufficiently sensitive to find it. The work of Robert Lowell, arguably the most important US poet of the last century, can be used to illustrate this point. The poem shown on page 43 does not refer to mood, but the fluency and richness of association it shows may originate in hypomania.

Second, psychiatric illness is stigmatizing. It takes courage to talk about these disorders, and this may be particularly true in a literary milieu, where there may be a good deal of denial that such illness is real, or there may be a vindictive desire to explain why it has happened in terms of the sufferer's personal relationships. Literary biography is often littered with fanciful explanation of why things turned out as they

Epilogue

Robert Lowell (1917–77)

Those blessèd structures, plot and rhyme –

why are they no help to me now

I want to make

something imagined, not recalled?

I hear the noise of my own voice:

The painter's vision is not a lens, it trembles to caress the light.

But sometimes everything I write

with the threadbare art of my eye

seems a snapshot,

lurid, rapid, garish, grouped,

heightened from life,

yet paralyzed by fact.

All's misalliance.

Yet why not say what happened?

Pray for the grace of accuracy

Vermeer gave to the sun's illumination

stealing like the tide across a map

to his girl solid with yearning.

We are poor passing facts,

warned by that to give

each figure in the photograph

his living name.

Reproduced with permission from *The Collected Poems of Robert Lowell*. Bidart R, Gewanter D (eds). London: Faber & Faber, 2003.

did, and is at its weakest when explaining away psychiatric illness. Sylvia Plath's husband, Ted Hughes, was subjected to remarkable criticism that implied he was responsible for her death by suicide, even though her diaries and her work show that her debilitating depressive states were recurrent from a time before they had met.

In our view, the failure to embrace and understand scientific accounts of mood disorder promotes stigma and superstition. We need reliable accounts of the world. Understanding that the Earth goes round the Sun does not make the sunrise less beautiful, but it does make it less likely that human sacrifices will be made to ensure it goes on happening.

Terminology and stigma

To reduce the stigma of mood disorders in general, and bipolar disorder in particular, champions are needed who can emerge from the closet and talk about what it is like to be affected. Because so many talented people have suffered from bipolar disorder, we do now have a literature of this sort.

William Styron has written rivetingly about the experience of depression and has pinpointed something that is beyond science, yet reflects on how we use and understand language:

> "Depression ... used to be termed melancholia ... 'Melancholia' would still appear to be a far more apt and evocative word for the blacker forms of the disorder, but it was usurped by a noun with a bland tonality and lacking any magisterial presence, used indifferently to describe an economic decline or a rut in the ground, a true wimp of a word."[3]

We certainly need to be alert to the nuances of terminology that do not ring true to patients; for example, the term bipolar is apparently preferred to 'manic-depressive' by many patients and is now used much more commonly.

It is questionable whether we should give in to more politicized attempts to change terminology. Such changes appear to arise from more totalitarian motives. A particular example is the very term 'patient'. We use the term patient because we find it to be widely understood and it places psychiatric patients on equal terms with patients with other diseases. Its original meaning – a sufferer – made

---

[3]From Styron W. *Darkness Visible. A Memoir of Madness.* New York: Random House, 1990.

Key points – the patient's perspective

- Mood disorder imposes extreme experiences on patients and their families, which are poorly appreciated by the general public and, too often perhaps, by clinicians.
- Mood disorder has played a central part in the lives of a disproportionate number of creative artists. Hypomania may lie at the core of extreme bursts of creative energy. Mania and depression contribute crucial experiences to the lives of creative artists, but madness is not the same as creativity.
- The patient's personal story is important to understanding the context and meaning of any illness.
- The scientific approach to diagnosis and treatment, which we unreservedly favor, is fully compatible with a humane and compassionate relationship with the patient.
- The relationship between mood disorder and creative experience is an important one, but states of frank mania or depression are rarely compatible with effective thought or action.

---

it a natural choice to describe those under medical care, at least for the last 600 years or so. The currently competing words are interesting.

- Client (from the Latin, originally describing the dependent relationship of a plebian to a patrician) is often deliberately used by psychologists and nurses to distinguish their relationship with patients from that of doctors. Quite how it incorporates a difference in practice or 'model', which is often implied, is not widely understood or, perhaps, understandable. The other connotations of the term client can be less satisfactory, conjuring up images of lawyers or prostitutes.
- The word consumer is more neutral, but implies a degree of choice many patients do not enjoy.
- The term user (of services) or service user is widely promoted, and even imposed, by current Department of Health policy in the UK. It reflects dissatisfaction with all references to illness or illness

connotations in 'Mental Health' services. Whether this denial of why we need such services at all will prove to be more or less stigmatizing is a moot point. If it proves inimical to a scientific approach to psychiatry, it will be a disaster.

We accept the key issue that clinicians must respect their patients as people who happen to have a mood disorder and never as diagnoses with an almost irrelevant human being attached. Good clinicians will hear their patients' stories and will understand some, at least, of the personal meanings these stories have, but they should not be seduced into thinking that this is ever enough. The best thing a doctor can do for his or her patient is to weigh the salience and reliability of information from history and examination in order to formulate an accurate diagnosis and offer appropriate treatment. This, together with a constructive therapeutic alliance, are essential elements in what we regard as the enhancement of care.

Key references

Caramagno T. *The Flight of the Mind*. Berkeley: University of California Press,1992. (A detailed account of Virginia Woolf's bipolar disorder.)

Jamison KR. *Touched with Fire: Manic-Depressive Illness and the Artistic Temperament*. New York and London: Simon & Schuster, 1994.

Jamison KR. *An Unquiet Mind. A Memoir of Moods and Madness*. London: Picador, 1996.

Lish JD, Dime-Meenan S, Whybrow PC et al. The National Depressive and Manic-Depressive Association (DMDA) survey of bipolar members. *J Affect Disord* 1994;31(4):281–94.

Lowell R. (Bidart F, Gewanter D, eds.) *The Collected Poems of Robert Lowell*. London: Faber & Faber, 2003.

Perlick D, Clarkin JF, Sirey J et al. Burden experienced by care-givers of persons with bipolar affective disorder. *Br J Psychiatry* 1999;175:56–62.

Styron W. *Darkness Visible. A Memoir of Madness*. New York: Random House, 1990.

Woolf V. *Mrs Dalloway*. Orlando, FL, USA: Harcourt, 1990. (First published by Hogarth Press, 1925.)

It makes sense to speak of enhancing care only if there is reason to think that the care being offered to bipolar patients is currently less than it should be. The basics, of course, never change: doctors should take a careful history, conduct a relevant physical examination and make the necessary investigations to formulate their diagnosis. This, and the medical plan of management, should be explained. Communication must be clear and effective. The objective is a therapeutic alliance between doctor and patient, which is always required for the management of a complex chronic condition.

Bipolar patients require more than this, because they must assume such a critical self-management role in an illness that can distort perception and judgement. They must acquire knowledge, experience and skill, and they need the help of their friends and relatives.

Knowledge (or 'psychoeducation')

Our patients must learn that their acute breakdowns are caused by the illness we call bipolar disorder. Mania and depression in the course of a bipolar illness are not simply understandable responses to stress or one-off problems that are unlikely to recur. Acceptance of these difficult facts is a key early objective of patient education.

Doctors, patients and carers usually start from different positions in building the therapeutic relationship. It is unsurprising that they make different estimates of future risks, since they bring different experiences and beliefs to the process. As already indicated, we believe that patients and carers need to know the facts, as currently distilled in the preceding chapters of this book. This is essential in order to address the seriousness of the illness, the high risk of relapse and the benefit of active treatment. We cannot expect a patient or carer to know what to do or to do it, unless they know why it may make a difference.

Clearly, there is no single way to teach effectively. The efficacy of a group or class was recently shown in a randomized controlled trial, but we favor a range of didactic teaching approaches, live or by video, written materials or guided Internet searching for high quality material (e.g. the National electronic Library for Mental Health, www.nelmh.org/ and Depression and Bipolar Support Alliance, www.dbsalliance.org). Educational efforts need to be sustained and progress is likely to be incremental. A shared and consistent approach across mental health disciplines is helpful, perhaps even essential.

Ultimately, there may be no substitute for experience, however bitter it may be. Doctors must be prepared to tolerate the repeated triumph of hope over experience before a patient finally becomes convinced of the need to take their self-management seriously.

The educational syllabus is effectively the content of this book. Clinicians and other healthcare workers should not be surprised or feel threatened by patients who appear to know, literally, more than they do. Patients will still need your help when it matters – when they become acutely ill – and they will respect you for not claiming to know everything. Patients, and their supporters as well, will benefit most from education delivered outside periods of acute episodes.

Skills

Once a patient accepts the broad facts about bipolar disorder, they give up a sense of personal responsibility for at least part of what the disorder is about. However, there is a new challenge, which is to identify and adjust those aspects of lifestyle and behavior that may be making things worse than they could and should be. Patients need to acquire new skills to manage their mood disorder as effectively as possible.

Patients must learn how to monitor and recognize relevant symptoms or signs and initiate an action plan. For example, sleep disturbance is the most frequently described final common pathway to mania. Shortening of the sleep cycle may be relatively easy to monitor and is susceptible to early treatment by social withdrawal or self-medication. Such early intervention implies patient autonomy. If the focus is sleep disturbance, the patient should keep a benzodiazepine or other hypnotic available. Antipsychotics may also be taken at the onset of a manic episode to reduce its severity. In addition, an increase in the dose of other medicines may be agreed under specific circumstances.

This gives the individual a greater sense of control, and permits immediate action. Other impulses and preoccupations may form part of the relatively stereotyped prodrome to relapse in individual patients. The involvement of family members may also be helpful, even essential, but must be treated sensitively, since it will not always be welcomed by the patient.

Patients may inadvertently risk relapse by irregular and even reckless patterns of activity and sleep. The establishment of routine and regular activity is thus a primary goal of treatment. Daily self-monitoring of mood, anxiety, activity and sleep forms a central component of most enhanced-care packages. Self-monitoring is employed in many psychological treatments and makes good intuitive sense to 40–60% of bipolar patients. Part of a mood chart form is shown in Figure 5.1 (blank forms with instructions for patients and clinicians can be downloaded at www.manicdepressive.org).

No treatment plan will work if alcohol or drug misuse is a significant problem. Abstinence must be an unambiguous goal in treatment for such patients.

The general point emerges that outcomes for patients can often be improved by simple, common-sense behavioral interventions. Translating this observation into enhanced care for more patients should be an important objective for treatment.

Family and friends

Community-based services impose appreciable burdens of responsibility and care on the family and friends of patients with bipolar disorder. The perceptions and beliefs that carers hold regarding bipolar disorder, as for other diseases, may have important effects on the levels of burden that are experienced. Perhaps unsurprisingly, it appears that accepting an illness model of the problem – rather than blaming the patient – reduces the carer's perception of stress.

Adherence to medicines

Patient outcomes can be improved by the measures described above for enhancing care, but this approach is not a substitute for long-term treatment with medicines. Moreover, no medicine can work if a patient

MOOD

Rate with 2 marks each day to indicate best and worst

0 = none
1 = mild
2 = moderate
3 = severe

Irritability	Anxiety	Hours Slept Last Night	Depressed — Severe: Significant Impairment NOT ABLE TO WORK	Depressed — Mod.: Significant Impairment ABLE TO WORK	Depressed — Mild: Without Significant Impairment	WNL — MOOD NOT DEFINITELY ELEVATED OR DEPRESSED. NO SYMPTOMS. Circle date to indicate Menses	Elevated — Mild: Without Significant Impairment	Elevated — Mod.: Significant Impairment ABLE TO WORK	Elevated — Severe: Significant Impairment NOT ABLE TO WORK	Psychotic Symptoms (Strange Ideas, Hallucinations)
2	1	7			X	X 1				
2	1	6		X		2 X				
2	1	8		X		X 3				
1	2	8				X 4	X			
1	2	8			X	X 5				
1	1	9		X	X	6				
1	2	9		X		X 7				
1	2	9		X		X 8				
1	2	9		X	X	9				
1	1	7		X		10 X				
1	1	7				11	X			
1	1	6			X	X 12				
1	1	7		X		X 13				
1	2	8			X	X 14				
2	1	8			X	X 15				
1	1	9			X	X 16				
1	1	6				17	X			
1	1	5			X	18		X		
1	1	6				19 X		X		
1	1	4				20	X		X	
2	2	6				21 X		X		
2	2	5				X 22		X		
2	2	8			X	23			X	
2	2	5				X 24		X		
2	2	6				25 X			X	
1	3	5				26	X	X		
2	2	9				X 27		X		
2	3	8			X	28 X				
1	2	7		X		X 29				
1	2	7			X	30 X				
						X 31 X				

Figure 5.1 Part of a mood chart for a rapid-cycling patient. This illustrates relative mood stability with an excess of depressive symptoms from day 1 to day 16, with a swing from day 17 to more elevated mood and greater instability.

fails to take it, and adherence (also known as compliance or, rarely, as concordance) is poor in many chronic illnesses. Bipolar disorder is no exception: non-adherence with treatment occurs in up to 50% of most clinical samples. Hence, adherence to prescribed medicines is a key issue.

Given the profiles of the existing medicines, it is often assumed that their adverse effects are a major reason for early discontinuation. Many such effects are subjective (e.g. tiredness and sedation), but no less important for that. Adverse effects should be minimized by dose adjustments, once-daily administration (e.g. at bedtime) and switching between formulations or comparable medicines. Generic prescribing is more difficult in psychiatry in general and mood disorder in particular, because of such complaints. The availability of a formulary, which offers a choice between different chemical entities of a similar class, is an important and necessary component of enhanced treatment.

Weight gain is a major long-term problem that merits greater prophylactic advice and planning than it usually receives. The monitoring of weight, glucose intolerance and cardiovascular risk factors should be a responsibility that the psychiatrist either undertakes or shares with a primary care physician or specialist.

The motivation to take tablets is not, however, determined simply by side effects. Especially in the long term, it also depends heavily on a knowledge of why the medicines are being prescribed, and the balance between cost and benefit perceived by patients and their carers. It is therefore not surprising that psychological interventions can improve adherence and, indeed, that this may account for a large part of the improved outcome associated with psychological approaches. This is illustrated in Figure 5.2.

Cognitive–behavior therapy

Cognitive–behavior therapy (CBT) is widely promoted as an approach to the treatment of mood disorder. It was developed from Beck's specific formulation of a cognitive model for depression. It emphasizes the potential for thoughts and memories to influence mood, rather than vice versa. Its focus is on conscious cognitive biases that may lead patients to

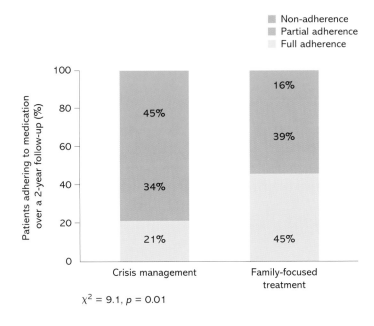

Non-adherence
Partial adherence
Full adherence

$\chi^2 = 9.1, p = 0.01$

Figure 5.2 Adherence to prescribed medicines can be improved by high-intensity psychological intervention to increase knowledge and family communication, compared with an approach oriented more to crisis management. (Reproduced with permission from Dr D Miklowitz.)

make negative interpretations of potentially neutral or even positive events or difficulties.

In its more refined forms (e.g. in relation to panic disorder), the treatment and its 'mechanism of action' are claimed to be specifically and optimally suited to the psychopathology of the patient's condition. For bipolar disorder, in which a cognitive component is only one of several probable contributing mechanisms, there can be little claim for specificity. CBT is instead a pragmatic approach to the problem that thoughts or beliefs may influence feelings.

As a time-limited and practical intervention, CBT occupies an emerging place in the management of bipolar disorder. Encouragingly, unlike other psychotherapists, CBT practitioners have always embraced the testing of efficacy by clinical trials. Results of the first trial of CBT for bipolar disorder suggest that it can help to achieve a modest reduction in relapse rates, especially in depression, and can improve adherence to medicines.

CBT has become a popular treatment option. However, psychotherapy is not always what it purports to be. Regulation is obviously more difficult than for a medicine. Some caution may therefore be required when seeking help, especially in the private sector. Patients should not be afraid to ask for proof of professional qualification and evidence of good practice.

Giving advice: functional impairments

Clinicians will be consulted about expectations and capacity to work. Major decisions should not normally be made by patients in a depressive or manic state. Judgment in depression may be excessively pessimistic, and in mania notoriously optimistic.

Even after recovery from an acute episode, patients may experience unexpected difficulty performing at a level appropriate to their education or training. This may be the consequence of common

---

Key points – enhanced care

- Enhancement of patient care is required to improve the capacity of patients to manage their bipolar disorder.
- Patients require knowledge and skills to realize this objective.
- Change can be achieved by structured interventions based on principles derived from behavioral and cognitive psychology.
- Abstinence from drugs and alcohol is necessary for effective treatment.
- The adoption of a disciplined and regular pattern of everyday activity is believed to facilitate mood stability.
- A key skill is to detect prodromes of illness by self-monitoring and implement an action plan appropriate to the developing risk.
- Adherence to prescribed medicines is an important objective of psychological treatment.
- Advising patients about decision-making and capacity to work is often an important part of the clinician's role.

sub-syndromal symptoms of depression or anxiety, or other barriers to psychological well-being. There may even be factors specific to bipolar disorder, such as experience when high, or personality style, that conspire to widen the gap between aspiration and achievement. Clinical input may be limited to encouragement and appropriate supportive letters, but is often important.

Rather differently, there is now consistent evidence that objective impairments of neuropsychological function are both significant and enduring in patients with bipolar I disorder. These changes appear to be acquired in the wake of recurrent episodes of illness and are evident initially as impairment in sustained attention. More extensive changes in cognitive function extending to memory and executive domains may be a later development. Our conviction is that, if these outcomes are avoidable with effective early treatment, then early diagnosis and management will assume increasing importance in the coming years.

Key references

American Psychiatric Association. Practice guideline for the treatment of patients with bipolar disorder (revision). *Am J Psychiatry* 2002;159(4 Suppl):1–50.

Colom F, Vieta E, Martinez-Aran A et al. Randomized trial on the efficacy of group psychoeducation in the prophylaxis of recurrences in remitted bipolar patients. *Arch Gen Psychiatry* 2003;60(4):402–7.

Horne R, Weinman J. Patients' beliefs about prescribed medicines and their role in adherence to treatment in chronic physical illness. *J Psychosom Res* 1999;47(6):555–67.

Johnson RE, McFarland BH. Lithium use and discontinuation in a health maintenance organization. *Am J Psychiatry* 1996;153(8):993–1000.

Lam D, Watkins E, Hayward P et al. A randomised controlled study of cognitive therapy of relapse prevention for bipolar affective disorder – outcome of the first year. *Arch Gen Psychiatry* 2003;60:145–152.

Leventhal H, Diefenbach M, Leventhal EA. Illness cognition: using common sense to understand treatment adherence and affect cognition interactions. *Cognit Ther Res* 1992;16(2):143–63.

Miklowitz DJ, George EL, Jeffrey A et al. A randomized study of family-focused psychoeducation and pharmacotherapy in the outpatient management of bipolar disorder. *Arch Gen Psychiatry* 2003;60:904–12.

Bipolar disorder often runs an episodic course and it is commonly thought of as a sequence of acute episodes of illness (mania, depression or mixed states) interspersed by euthymia. Short-term treatments are used in acute episodes, with the intention of discontinuing the medication on recovery. Long-term treatments are indefinite and are intended to prevent new episodes.

This simplified view of the illness is convenient and reflects how trials have been designed. However, sub-syndromal and chronic symptoms are common in bipolar disorder, and it is important to be aware of them. Chronic symptoms are usually depressive and are a disabling aspect of the long-term outcome. Unfortunately, there is little to guide the selection of treatment for these important clinical states. What we can be certain about is based on trials in bipolar I disorder and addresses syndrome-level morbidity.

Treatment options for mania and mixed states

Mania is often a medical emergency and carries appreciable risk for patients and those who are close to them. There are no reliable alternatives to treatment with medicines of proven efficacy. However, admission to hospital is itself associated with a subsequent fall in the level of symptoms. There are few specific measures that are recommended for the management of patients with mania and the most appropriate ward milieu has not been empirically established. Common sense suggests that a calming, uncrowded environment without over-stimulation is likely to be best.

Figure 6.1 shows a flow chart derived from recommendations in the British Association for Psychopharmacology (BAP) guidelines on the treatment of bipolar disorder. It outlines a simplified decision tree for mania and mixed episodes. The options are described in detail below. Drugs used in short-term treatment of acute mania and mixed states are summarized in Table 6.1.

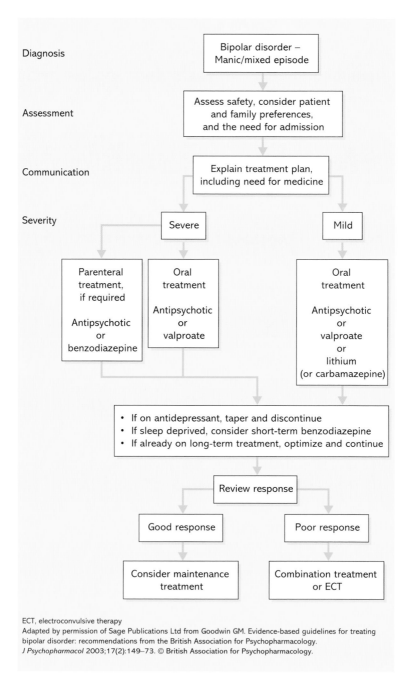

ECT, electroconvulsive therapy
Adapted by permission of Sage Publications Ltd from Goodwin GM. Evidence-based guidelines for treating
bipolar disorder: recommendations from the British Association for Psychopharmacology.
J Psychopharmacol 2003;17(2):149–73. © British Association for Psychopharmacology.

Figure 6.1 Initial treatment scheme – mania and mixed states.

TABLE 6.1

Drugs used in the short-term treatment of acute mania and mixed states

Class	Drug	Dose for uncompromised adult* (daily dose unless otherwise stated)
Typical antipsychotics (avoid EPS)	Chlorpromazine	• Orally: 300–1000 mg, as tablets, syrup or suspension • Intramuscular: 50 mg every 6–8 hours • Per rectum: 100 mg every 6–8 hours
	Haloperidol	• Oral: 3–10 mg, as tablets or liquid • Intramuscular (or intravenous): 2–10 mg every 8 hours • Depot: 50–100 mg per month (as decanoate)
Atypical antipsychotics	Olanzapine	• Oral: 10–20 mg as tablets or oro-dispersible • Intramuscular: 5–10 mg (20 mg maximum) as up to 3 injections per 24 hours
	Risperidone	• Oral: 3–6 mg as tablets or liquid • Depot: 25–50 mg every 2 weeks
	Quetiapine	• Oral: 200–800 mg as tablets, taper in (average dose 600 mg)
	Ziprasidone	• Oral: 80–160 mg as tablets • Intramuscular: 10–20 mg every 4 hours (to a maximum of 40 mg)
	Aripiprazole	• Oral: 10–15 mg as tablets
	Clozapine	• Oral: 100–800 mg, taper in as tolerated, tablets
Anticonvulsants	Valproate	• Oral: 750–1250 mg as semi-sodium, tablets; increase by 30% for sodium valproate
	Carbamazepine	• Oral: taper up to 1200 mg, tablets
	Oxcarbazepine	• Oral: taper up to 1200 mg, tablets
Lithium	Lithium carbonate (note formulations have different bioavailability)	• Oral: 400–1200 mg as tablets, 500–300 mg as liquid, according to blood level (> 1 and < 1.5 mmol/L for mania)
	Lithium citrate	• Oral: as liquid 500–3000 mg, according to blood level

(CONTINUED)

57

TABLE 6.1 (CONTINUED)

Class	Drug	Dose for uncompromised adult* (daily dose unless otherwise stated)
Benzodiazepines	Lorazepam	• Oral: 4–16 mg in divided doses, tablets • Intravenous: 2–4 mg every 6–8 hours, slowly into a large vein
	Clonazepam	• Oral: 2–8 mg in divided doses, tablets • Intravenous: 1 mg every 6–8 hours, slowly into a large vein

*Reduce dose in the elderly or if otherwise indicated
EPS, extrapyramidal side effects

Antipsychotics. Mania has long been treated with antipsychotic medicines. Indeed, at the start of the psychotropic era, chlorpromazine was first used with patients who had manic psychoses as well as schizophrenia. However, the efficacy of the older, so-called typical, antipsychotics was never examined in placebo-controlled trials. Instead, the short-term effect of acute tranquilization was probably taken to be self-evident. Indeed, the old term 'major tranquilizer' betrays the effect that was sought through sedation and even motor side effects – some clinicians used to refer approvingly to a 'chemical straitjacket'. Inevitably, such effects have often been associated with high doses and consequent severe adverse effects.

Pragmatic support for the use of an antipsychotic agent rather than lithium in severe mania came from a secondary analysis of data comparing generous doses of chlorpromazine and lithium. This suggested that the most activated manic patients were more effectively treated with chlorpromazine. The outcomes were realistic measures, such as the patient dropout rate and reduced nursing demands. Clinical practice has also tended to support the use of antipsychotics.

Antipsychotics are not merely sedative, they are also antimanic. This has been established by the results of recent trials examining the efficacy of the so-called atypical antipsychotics. The atypicals have a primary mode of action that is probably via blockade of dopamine receptors, although it remains controversial as to how the risk of extrapyramidal side effects (EPS) is reduced. It is a reasonable hypothesis that mania is a hyper-dopaminergic state and that blockade of dopamine receptors represents an appropriate approach to treatment. Certainly, trials with olanzapine, ziprasidone, aripiprazole, quetiapine and risperidone now support the efficacy of atypical antipsychotics as a class in mania. Olanzapine and ziprasidone[1] are available in a parenteral formulation for acute use and risperidone is available as a long-acting injectable formulation.

Data from seminal studies with olanzapine are shown in Figure 6.2. Olanzapine was found to be superior to placebo (in two trials) and

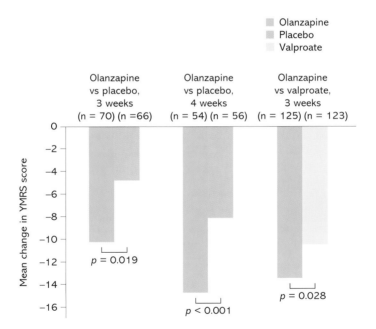

Figure 6.2 Summary of data from three seminal studies with olanzapine. The average treatment effects are shown as the mean reduction in score on the Young Mania Rating Scale (YMRS) for olanzapine vs placebo for 3 weeks and for 4 weeks, and olanzapine vs valproate for 3 weeks. In each trial, olanzapine was shown to be significantly superior to the comparator.

---

[1]Ziprasidone is not available in the UK.

also, though more marginally, to valproate. The reduction in the Young Mania Rating Scale is presented as a global effect, but change occurred on almost every item of the scale and not preferentially on those related to sedation. Olanzapine has also been shown to have comparable efficacy to haloperidol.

EPS are manifest as akathisia, parkinsonism or dystonia during acute treatment, and patients with bipolar disorder are probably more likely to show acute EPS when treated with comparable doses of haloperidol than those with schizophrenia. There are two important clinical disadvantages to this. First, the subjective experience of EPS, especially akathisia and dystonia, may be highly aversive and produce a negative attitude in patients towards subsequent treatment of their illness with any sort of medicine. Second, naturalistic studies in schizophrenia suggest that development of acute EPS is predictive of subsequent tardive dyskinesia. The most important clinical message is simply that antimanic action can be achieved without EPS and the improved therapeutic ratio of the atypical antipsychotics makes it easier to treat mania without inducing EPS.

There is increasing international support for the use of antipsychotics as first-line agents for mania and this is reflected by the advice contained in a number of recent guidelines.

Valproate, lithium and carbamazepine. The seminal randomized, placebo-controlled trial of valproate in acute mania in the 1990s was the catalyst for major changes in the treatment of bipolar disorder. This trial not only showed that valproate is an effective antimanic agent, but also that lithium appears to have comparable efficacy. Valproate is a generic term used to describe the several formulations of valproic acid, which is the presumed active chemical entity. Sodium valproate is widely used in epilepsy and is available as a sustained-release preparation. Valproate semisodium (divalproex in North America) is a non-covalent dimer molecule that has been produced in several formulations (best known as Depakote), including a slow-release form. In bipolar disorder, valproate has been studied almost exclusively as valproate semisodium. Valproate is effective in severe (including psychotic) mania. Aggressive dosing to achieve serum levels effective against mania (> 80 µg/dL) may result in acute gastrointestinal side effects, sedation or cognitive impairment, but it does not produce EPS.

Lithium was initially discovered to be an antimanic agent by Cade in 1947, but early trials did not employ modern methodology, such as parallel group design, formal rating scales and statistical analysis. Lithium monotherapy is generally preferred for the treatment of less severe manic states.

There is also limited evidence to support the efficacy of carbamazepine in mania, but it is seldom advocated as first-line treatment. Oxcarbazepine is a distinct but related chemical entity with a somewhat reduced potential for pharmacokinetic interactions. Its efficacy has not been established.

Other drugs. Gabapentin, lamotrigine and topiramate have been examined in acute mania and found to be ineffective. Unproven and ineffective treatments are not acceptable alternatives to those agents shown to be effective treatments for acute mania in randomized controlled trials.

Combination treatment. Many episodes of mania occur in patients who are already taking lithium or valproate as a long-term treatment. In such cases, it is common to continue lithium or valproate and add an antipsychotic. This strategy is supported by trials in which risperidone, haloperidol, olanzapine and also quetiapine in combination with lithium or valproate have proved superior to monotherapy with lithium or valproate alone.

These findings underpin the current advice of the American Psychiatric Association, which also recommends combining lithium or valproate with an antipsychotic in patients who are not already receiving long-term treatment. It clearly makes sense when there is reason to spare the antipsychotic dose and/or long-term treatment with lithium or valproate is planned. However, adherence is such a major issue that the initiation of long-term treatment when patients are manic may not be a good strategy unless the attitude of the patient when well is already known.

Carbamazepine is not an ideal agent for combination treatment because liver enzyme induction may reduce the levels of other drugs. Oxcarbazepine may overcome this disadvantage.

Benzodiazepines are not believed to be antimanic. They are used as an adjunct to other agents and may be required when sedation or tranquilization is a priority (e.g. after a prolonged period of sleep deprivation). Benzodiazepines are safe and have few important pharmacokinetic interactions with other agents. Their use may also reduce the required doses of antipsychotics or other drugs.

Strategy for treating mania

The objective in treating mania is to control behavioral disturbance and shorten the duration of the episode. Where possible, the treatment should be agreed with the patient and thought should be given to the creation of advance directives, which may facilitate future treatment. Antipsychotics or valproate, as monotherapy or in combination, are the preferred options. However, avoidance of EPS is also a priority. This argues for minimal doses of classical antipsychotics if used, a low threshold for the use of valproate or atypical antipsychotics, and careful monitoring of clinical response. Restoration of the sleep/wake cycle, if greatly disturbed, is an early objective.

Benzodiazepines should be withdrawn once their desired effect on sleep has been obtained. Antipsychotic agents should be continued until full remission of acute symptoms has been achieved (up to 2–3 months). There should be an early emphasis on understanding the patient's attitude to treatment in the long term and clinicians must be aware of the risk of a switch to depression. It is not established which treatments, if any, make such a switch more likely.

Short-term treatments and mixed states

Mixed states may be slower to resolve during acute treatment than more classic mania. There have been no studies to determine the optimal treatment for this subgroup by comparison with other manic presentations. Secondary analyses of subgroups of patients with mixed states suggest that combination therapy with olanzapine and valproate or lithium is particularly effective. However, in common with most such analyses, they may be misleading because sample sizes are under-powered. There is no reason to start or continue treatment with an antidepressant in a mixed state where the predominant effect is manic.

Electroconvulsive therapy (ECT) in refractory mania and mixed states. Audit studies suggest that ECT is a highly effective treatment for mania, with response rates of over 80%. Given its established effects on severe depression, ECT might also be expected to work well in mixed states. However, there are no randomized, controlled trials to support the use ECT in mania or mixed states. It is clearly an option for those patients who express a preference for it, when mania is refractory to drug treatment and in those with severe mania during pregnancy, when drug treatment may be undesirable. It is of course more usual for ECT to be considered for the treatment of depression in bipolar patients.

Treatment options for depressive episodes
Patients with bipolar disorder will, on average, spend more of their time depressed than in manic or mixed states. It is surprising, therefore, that the treatment of bipolar depression has been very neglected over many years and there is a paucity of randomized evidence to demonstrate the efficacy or relative effectiveness of different approaches in relieving depressive symptoms.

Figure 6.3 shows a flow chart derived from recommendations in the BAP guideline for the treatment of bipolar depressive episodes. Table 6.2 lists drugs used in the short-term treatment of acute depressive states. The options are described below in more detail.

Antidepressants. Compared with the evidence for the effectiveness of antidepressants in unipolar disorder, the available data relating specifically to bipolar depression is extremely limited. Overall, the existing data on a variety of different antidepressants (imipramine, fluoxetine and tranylcypromine) favor a benefit compared with placebo, whether or not they are added to a mood stabilizer. The audit of outcomes of patients admitted to hospital with unipolar and bipolar disorder supports the view that both are responsive to treatment with tricyclic antidepressants (TCAs). An

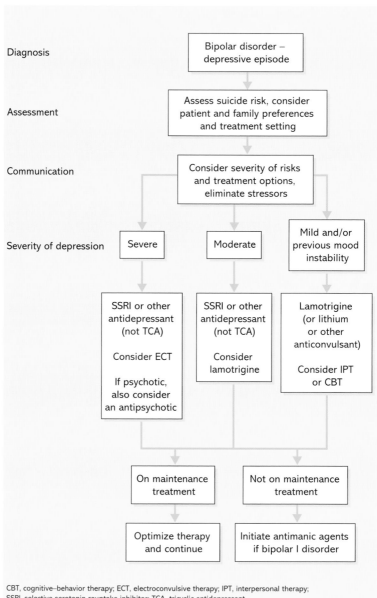

Diagnosis → Bipolar disorder – depressive episode

Assessment → Assess suicide risk, consider patient and family preferences and treatment setting

Communication → Consider severity of risks and treatment options, eliminate stressors

Severity of depression → Severe | Moderate | Mild and/or previous mood instability

Severe: SSRI or other antidepressant (not TCA). Consider ECT. If psychotic, also consider an antipsychotic

Moderate: SSRI or other antidepressant (not TCA). Consider lamotrigine

Mild and/or previous mood instability: Lamotrigine (or lithium or other anticonvulsant). Consider IPT or CBT

On maintenance treatment → Optimize therapy and continue

Not on maintenance treatment → Initiate antimanic agents if bipolar I disorder

CBT, cognitive–behavior therapy; ECT, electroconvulsive therapy; IPT, interpersonal therapy; SSRI, selective serotonin reuptake inhibitor; TCA, tricyclic antidepressant
Adapted by permission of Sage Publications Ltd from Goodwin GM. Evidence-based guidelines for treating bipolar disorder: recommendations from the British Association for Psychopharmacology. *J Psychopharmacol* 2003;17(2):149–73. © British Association for Psychopharmacology.

Figure 6.3 Initial treatment scheme – bipolar depressive episode.

TABLE 6.2

Drugs used in the short-term treatment of acute depressive states

Class	Drug	Daily dose for uncompromised adult*
Antidepressants: SSRIs	Citalopram	20–60 mg as tablets or oral drops
	Escitalopram (isomer)	10–20 mg as tablets
	Sertraline	100–200 mg as tablets
	Fluoxetine	10–20 mg as tablets or liquid
	Paroxetine	20–50 mg as tablets or liquid
	Fluvoxamine	100–300 mg as tablets
Antidepressants: other	Bupropion	150–300 mg as tablets
Antidepressants: MAOIs	Moclobemide	300–600 mg as tablets
	Tranylcypromine	10–20 mg as tablets
	Phenelzine	30–75 mg as tablets
Lithium	See Table 6.1	Choose level > 0.5 mmol/L, according to tolerability
Anticonvulsants	Lamotrigine	100–400 mg as tablets, tapered in slowly (see package insert)
	Valproate	See Table 6.1: little to guide dosing
Atypical antipsychotics	Olanzapine	See Table 6.1

*Reduce dose in the elderly or if otherwise indicated
MAOIs, monoamine oxidase inhibitors; SSRIs, selective serotonin reuptake inhibitors

important caveat, however, relates to the increased risk of a switch to mania with TCAs.

There are no grounds at present for recommending one antidepressant over another on the basis of efficacy.

Antidepressants are best used in combination with an agent that will reduce the risk of mania (lithium, valproate or an antipsychotic).

ECT is effective in severe depression and the randomized trials of ECT have included bipolar cases, although there have been no studies that have concentrated exclusively on bipolar groups. A recent, systematic review of ECT supports its general efficacy and also its relatively greater efficacy compared with antidepressants. The adverse consequence of memory disturbance may not be dissociable from effective dosing, but is usually mild. The use of ECT is tempered by the continuing unfavorable portrayal of the treatment by the media, and anecdotal reports of very severe, but largely unexplained, subjective side effects such as loss of identity, complete amnesia and inability to read. The most extravagant claims about the adverse effects of ECT appear less likely to be due to the treatment than to other grievances in the minds of the claimants. Access to ECT will continue to be necessary, because it offers such an effective way of relieving very severe and dangerous depressive states.

Lithium. Evidence for the acute efficacy of lithium in bipolar depression is generally inadequate; early trials were all small crossover studies of short duration. It is also emerging from systematic review of the trials of long-term treatment that the efficacy of lithium in preventing depressive relapse is also modest, and less than its efficacy against mania. Nevertheless, lithium occupies a prominent place in many treatment guidelines, which express expert preference for the use of lithium, rather than antidepressants, as first-line treatment for bipolar depression. The conflict between opinion and evidence highlights an area of considerable uncertainty. It would be helpful if lithium is included as a key comparator in new monotherapy studies of compounds developed for use specifically in bipolar disorder.

Anticonvulsants. Because of their reputation as 'mood stabilizers', the anticonvulsants carbamazepine and valproate are also often advocated for use in acute depression, although the evidence supporting their efficacy is almost non-existent. Lamotrigine, which has an entirely different mechanism of action, is the only anticonvulsant compound for which there is evidence supporting a significant clinical benefit in acute bipolar depression. It does not increase the risk of switching.

Antipsychotics have long had a place in the management of psychotic depression, but their more routine use in the treatment of bipolar depression is an emerging development. Olanzapine appears to be a modest antidepressant in bipolar depression, but has a greater effect when combined with fluoxetine. The serotonergic actions of some of the atypical antipsychotics may make them unusually efficacious in depressed states.

Mania following depression

Just like the switch from mania to depression, a switch from depression to mania may be a consequence either of the course of the illness or of the treatment; some treatments may have a greater propensity to cause switching than others. Both in practice and in theory, it is difficult to disentangle whether or not mania has been triggered by drug treatment. Only randomized, placebo-controlled trials of monotherapy can establish whether certain drugs increase the probability of switching, and most trials of this design are short-term, which reduces the time during which such a switch may be observed. Meta-analysis has shown that a manic event is 2–3 times more likely to occur during treatment with TCAs than during treatment with selective serotonin reuptake inhibitors (SSRIs) or placebo. Coadministration of an antimanic agent can, however, reduce this risk.

Strategy for treating depression

It is usually recommended that antidepressants be discontinued after the acute resolution of symptoms. This reflects a belief that antidepressants tend to destabilize the course of the illness in bipolar patients (see above). It appears to be true when patients cycle rapidly, since this may be reduced in a minority of cases by stopping an apparently provoking antidepressant. Whether the risk-to-benefit ratio is the same for all patients is less certain, especially when antidepressants are used in combination with antimanic agents. When antidepressants are discontinued, it is recommended that the dose should be tapered off over 4 weeks, if possible. Antidepressants may be discontinued more quickly if patients develop mania.

Refractory depression is not uncommon. There is no specific recommendation for bipolar disorder, and treatment should follow recommendations for refractory depression in general.

It remains uncertain whether the treatment of depression in patients with bipolar spectrum disorder should be different from the treatment in patients with unipolar disorder.

Key points – short-term treatments

- The objective of short-term treatment is to reduce the severity and shorten the duration of an acute episode.
- Antipsychotics, valproate and lithium are antimanic. The clinical context and, whenever possible, patient preference and experience should determine the choice.
- Antipsychotics may be preferred in highly active or agitated patients with mania. Extrapyramidal side effects (EPS) are unnecessary for treatment efficacy and should, if possible, be avoided. Valproate is also effective in severe mania.
- The atypical antipsychotics (olanzapine, ziprasidone, aripiprazole, quetiapine and risperidone) have shown efficacy as monotherapy in placebo-controlled trials in mania and are less likely to produce EPS.
- Combining an antipsychotic with lithium or valproate can facilitate the acute treatment response. Combinations with risperidone, haloperidol, olanzapine or quetiapine have been shown to be superior to lithium or valproate alone, especially when mania recurs on maintenance therapy.
- Benzodiazepines can induce sedation or regularize sleep when added to antimanic agents. They should be discontinued after the desired response is established.
- Short-term treatments for mania can be discontinued after full remission of symptoms (usually 2–3 months).

(CONTINUED)

- A switch from mania to depression may occur in any illness course and it is not established which treatments, if any, make this more likely.
- Electroconvulsive therapy provides an important treatment option for manic or mixed states resistant to treatment or arising in pregnancy, and for severe depression.
- Antidepressants are effective for treating depression in bipolar disorder, but are best used in combination with an agent that will reduce the risk of mania (lithium, valproate or possibly an antipsychotic).
- The risk of a switch from depression to mania is greater with tricyclic antidepressants than with other antidepressants (particularly selective serotonin reuptake inhibitors).
- Lamotrigine probably has acute efficacy in depression, without a risk of inducing switching.
- The discontinuation of antidepressants is currently recommended after remission of an acute episode of depression.

Key references

Bhagwagar Z, Goodwin GM. The role of lithium in the treatment of bipolar depression. *Clin Neurosci Res* 2002;2:222–7.

Bottlender R, Rudolf D, Strauss A, Moller HJ. Mood-stabilisers reduce the risk of developing antidepressant-induced maniform states in acute treatment of bipolar I depressed patients. *J Affect Disord* 2001; 63(1–3):79–83.

Bowden CL, Brugger AM, Swann AC et al. Efficacy of divalproex vs lithium and placebo in the treatment of mania. *JAMA* 1994;271(12):918–24.

Gijsman HJ, Geddes JR, Rendell JM et al. Antidepressants for bipolar depression: a systematic review of randomised controlled trials. *Am J Psych* 2004 (in press)

Goodwin GM. Evidence-based guidelines for treating bipolar disorder: recommendations from the British Association for Psychopharmacology. *J Psychopharmacol* 2003;17: 149–73.

Mukherjee S, Sackeim HA, Schnur DB. Electroconvulsive therapy of acute manic episodes: a review of 50 years' experience. *Am J Psychiatry* 1994;151(2):169–76.

Muller-Oerlinghausen B, Retzow A, Henn FA et al. Valproate as an adjunct to neuroleptic medication for the treatment of acute episodes of mania: a prospective, randomized, double-blind, placebo-controlled, multicenter study. *J Clin Psychopharmacol* 2000;20(2):195–203.

Peet M. Induction of mania with selective serotonin re-uptake inhibitors and tricyclic antidepressants. *Br J Psychiatry* 1994;164(4):549–50.

Prien RF, Caffey E-M Jr, Klett CJ. Comparison of lithium carbonate and chlorpromazine in the treatment of mania. Report of the Veterans Administration and National Institute of Mental Health Collaborative Study Group. *Arch Gen Psychiatry* 1972;26(2):146–53.

Sachs GS, Grossman F, Ghaemi SN et al. Combination of a mood stabilizer with risperidone or haloperidol for treatment of acute mania: a double-blind, placebo-controlled comparison of efficacy and safety. *Am J Psychiatry* 2002;159(7):1146–54.

Sachs GS, Printz DJ, Kahn DA et al. The Expert Consensus Guideline Series: medication treatment of bipolar disorder 2000. *Postgrad Med* 2000;Spec No:1–104.

Tohen M, Jacobs TG, Grundy SL et al. Efficacy of olanzapine in acute bipolar mania: a double-blind, placebo-controlled study. *Arch Gen Psychiatry* 2000;57(9):841–9.

The UK ECT Review Group. Electroconvulsive therapy – systematic review and meta-analysis of efficacy and safety in depressive disorders. *Lancet* 2003;361: 799–808.

The objective of long-term treatment in bipolar disorder is to reduce the risk of relapse, suicide and overall mortality. This can also be referred to as mood stabilization, and drugs with efficacy against both manic and depressive relapse are often described as mood stabilizers.

The term mood stabilizer is a functional one that conveniently describes a group of otherwise pharmacologically different agents, rather like the term antipsychotic or antidepressant. Unfortunately, it has been bestowed indiscriminately on some anticonvulsants, such as gabapentin and topiramate, with little evidence to support efficacy against relapse. By contrast, the atypical antipsychotic olanzapine has been shown to prevent relapse and therefore is a mood stabilizer. In fact, the long-term use of a variety of agents alone or in combination may contribute to mood stability. More neutral terminology often seems prudent.

In unipolar disorder, relapse (the return of symptoms treated in an acute episode) is often distinguished from recurrence (the re-appearance of symptoms after the sustained remission of an index episode). This distinction is not useful in bipolar disorder, where episodes are often frequent. We will therefore refer to long-term treatment for prevention of relapse.

Figure 7.1 shows the long-term treatment scheme based on the British Association for Psychopharmacology guidelines. The main medications used in long-term management of bipolar disorder are listed in Table 7.1 (see page 80), together with some of the issues relating to safety.

Long-term treatment with lithium

Lithium is the classical long-term treatment for bipolar I disorder. There have been adequate, but not large, numbers of patients entered into placebo-controlled trials. Over 1 year, relapse rates in patients receiving lithium were 40% compared with 61% in those receiving placebo, and the relative risk reduction remains constant at 33% over 2–3 years. Patients who do well on lithium for this time period appear to continue to do well in the longer term.

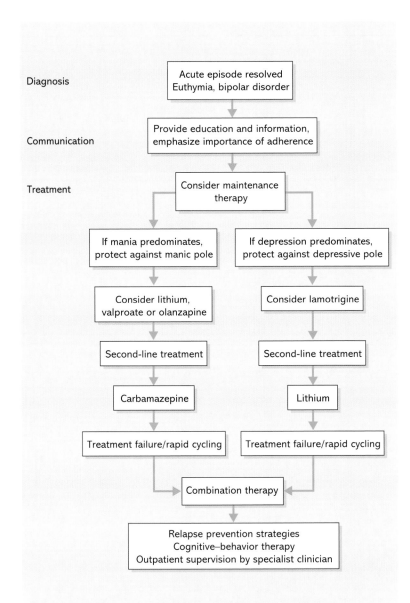

Adapted by permission of Sage Publications Ltd from Goodwin GM. Evidence-based guidelines for treating bipolar disorder: recommendations from the British Association for Psychopharmacology. *J Psychopharmacol* 2003;17(2):149–73. © British Association for Psychopharmacology.

Figure 7.1 Long-term treatment scheme – maintenance therapy.

In the prevention of relapse, lithium is probably more effective against mania than against depression (relative risk reduction of 40% vs 23%, respectively). Plasma lithium levels below 0.5 mmol/L are usually too low to be effective and levels over 0.8 mmol/L are often recommended. However, achieving high levels in the face of significant side effects is likely to be counterproductive. The highest dose that produces minimal side effects should be employed.

Long-term treatment with anticonvulsants

Anticonvulsants are often described quite uncritically as mood stabilizers. In part, this reflects the hypothesis that they work against an underlying 'instability' that has something in common with epilepsy. While this concept is heuristically useful, it is unlikely to be true. Anticonvulsants prevent seizures, but there is no evidence that they reverse the primary neuronal instability in epilepsy.

Valproate has been studied in a single, long-term, randomized, controlled trial, which was underpowered for its primary endpoint. Rates of relapse were 24% for valproate (as valproate semisodium) and 38% for placebo. While the difference is not statistically significant, it suggests a relative risk reduction of 37%, which is numerically comparable with lithium. It is not possible to say whether valproate has a greater efficacy against manic than against depressive relapse.

Despite this statistically weak evidence base, valproate is widely used in North America and increasingly used in other countries. It has a reputation for greater tolerability than lithium – certainly when lithium is used at doses that produce plasma levels over 0.8 mmol/L. However, it is not without adverse effects.

Carbamazepine was the first anticonvulsant to be advocated for the long-term treatment of bipolar disorder. However, it has been shown to be inferior to lithium in preventing relapse.

Lamotrigine has a novel profile in relapse prevention. It is more effective against depression than mania. Two long-term trials have compared lithium and lamotrigine with placebo, one in patients with a recent depressive episode and the other in patients with a recent manic episode. The findings were essentially the same in both studies. Overall, the benefit was similar for lithium and lamotrigine, but the largest effect of lithium was on manic relapse and the greatest effect of lamotrigine was on depression.

Long-term treatment with antipsychotics

Classical antipsychotics have often been used in bipolar patients as a long-term treatment, sometimes in depot formulations. Their place is poorly established, however, because of very limited evidence from clinical trials and concerns about tardive dyskinesia.

The atypical antipsychotics are currently the subject of intense study. Companies seeking to extend their product licenses for the treatment of schizophrenia to bipolar disorder are providing a mass of new data. Olanzapine is the best studied atypical agent to date. It has been shown to be effective in the long-term in a placebo-controlled study of relapse prevention in acute olanzapine responders. It also appears to be superior to lithium as monotherapy after an acute response to the combination of lithium with olanzapine. Like lithium, olanzapine appears to be more effective in preventing manic relapse than depressive relapse.

Antipsychotic agents may often be appropriate for the long-term management of bipolar patients, especially those in whom psychotic features are prominent. In addition, clozapine, used in combination with 'usual treatment' with lithium or anticonvulsants, has been shown to be superior to 'usual treatment' alone over 1 year in patients with treatment-resistant bipolar disorder, including those with rapid cycling and mixed states.

Long-term treatment with antidepressants

Antidepressant monotherapy is not recommended in patients with bipolar I disorder. A small but highly regarded study conducted more than 20 years ago cast a negative perspective on long-term antidepressant treatment. First, it showed that imipramine alone resulted in an unacceptable number of manic relapses over a 1–2-year follow-up period; this effect was prevented by cotreatment with lithium. Second, the combination of imipramine with lithium was only a little more effective than lithium alone in preventing depressive relapse. It remains uncertain whether or not antidepressants should be used long term in bipolar disorder, even in conjunction with other agents, because there have been no systematic large-scale studies to clarify the issue since this initial study. Given the significant burden of disease imposed by chronic depressive symptoms and recurrent depressive episodes, this may appear surprising.

The long-term treatment of bipolar I disorder with antidepressants is, however, common in clinical practice. Audit evidence generally supports successful long-term prophylaxis with antidepressants in bipolar patients who are also receiving lithium, valproate, carbamazepine or antipsychotics.

Patients with bipolar II disorder and, in particular, those with bipolar spectrum depression, have not been sufficiently investigated. It is possible that effective treatment with antidepressants can be achieved without an added antimanic agent. This area merits further investigation, as the diagnostic issues become more clearly defined.

Long-term combination therapy

The early discovery of lithium and its initial status as something of a 'wonder drug' perhaps exaggerated our perceptions of effectiveness of monotherapy with lithium. In fact, no more than 30% of patients started on lithium do well over a 5-year follow-up period. It has been a principle in other areas of medicine that the combination of two partially effective treatments may make a potent treatment. The same approach is now developing in bipolar disorder. In our view, it would be preferable to base practice on systematic audit and, preferably, randomized trials of particular combinations. Combination treatment can too quickly become bizarre polypharmacy.

Systematic study of combinations of currently available medicines appears increasingly necessary because of the intensifying pressure to intervene early in the natural history of bipolar disorder. Effective prevention of disease progression may require combination therapy from as early in the illness course as possible. We are uncertain what combination, if any, to recommend after a first episode. To resolve the key uncertainties, there is widespread support for large simple trials in bipolar disorder. Such trials require the creation of adequate capacity in the form of collaborative networks of clinicians who can incorporate simple trial methodology into everyday clinical practice.

Suicide

Suicide is a major long-term risk for patients with bipolar I disorder and contributes disproportionately to their increased mortality. Suicide rates are around 10% in the long-term follow-up of patients identified by admission to hospital – the most severely affected group. Suicide is associated with depression and mixed states. Therefore, successful long-term treatment has the potential to reduce the risk of suicide by preventing new episodes or reducing chronic symptoms. Naturalistic studies suggest that suicide rates are lower in patients who receive long-term treatment. Furthermore, lithium may have particular efficacy as an anti-suicide agent. This is supported by new evidence that valproate – although now more commonly initiated for long-term treatment than lithium in the USA – is not effective in reducing suicide rates while, in the same patient population, lithium is.

Stopping long-term treatment

Discontinuation of long-term treatment is not indicated when there is good clinical control of the illness. When necessary, it should be tapered, especially in the case of lithium, where there is a specific risk of manic relapse. Poor compliance is a contraindication to prescribing lithium because of the risk of new illness episodes on discontinuation.

Adverse effects of long-term treatment

Adverse effects certainly contribute to poor adherence to prescribed treatment and may pose dangers in their own right. Weight gain is the most important problem associated with many of the long-term drug treatments. It contributes to an increased risk of type 2 diabetes. In addition, there is concern that antipsychotics may increase the risk of diabetes by other, as yet poorly understood, mechanisms.

Tardive dyskinesia remains a concern for patients treated with long-term antipsychotics. Development of acute EPS appears to predict an increased risk of tardive dyskinesia and bipolar patients may be at a slightly greater risk of motor side effects when taking antipsychotics than are patients with schizophrenia.

Avoidance of EPS is an indication to use atypical antipsychotics, because they have a more favorable therapeutic ratio than classical antipsychotics. There are also differences between the atypical antipsychotics: for example, quetiapine and clozapine have an intrinsically lower capacity to occupy dopamine receptors than olanzapine and risperidone; increasing the dose of olanzapine and risperidone will produce motor effects, while increasing the dose of quetiapine and clozapine will not.

There is a related concern about prolactin elevation with some antipsychotics, especially those with high affinity for dopamine D2 receptors. This has long been associated with the typical antipsychotics, but is also seen with risperidone, for example, especially at higher doses. Hyperprolactinemia produces a hypogonadal state, which is most marked in women. Antipsychotics with a lower affinity for D2 receptors, such as clozapine and quetiapine, and the partial agonist aripiprazole are less likely to cause such problems in long-term treatment.

Prescribing in pregnancy and after childbirth

One of the more potent reasons for stopping long-term treatment arises when a woman with bipolar disorder wishes to become, or is already, pregnant. The decision of whether or not to stop treatment is reached by balancing clinical priorities, and will depend on the patient's preferences and past history. There is therefore no simple rule.

The potential benefits of compliance with long-term treatment during pregnancy are that the patient remains symptom-free and enjoys normal bonding with the child. However, cohort studies indicate that exposure to lithium, valproate or carbamazepine in the first 2 months of pregnancy increases the risk of major congenital malformations over the 2–4% risk seen in the general population. Lamotrigine and the antipsychotics generally appear to be safer.

On the other hand, withdrawal of medication may lead to relapse, which might harm the mother–child relationship directly or via comorbid alcohol, drug and nicotine consumption.

Treatment options include continuing existing medications throughout pregnancy, switching to alternatives associated with lower

Key points – long-term treatments

- Long-term treatment with appropriate drugs is advocated from as early in the illness as is acceptable to the patient and family.
- The term mood stabilizer is likely to be bestowed increasingly liberally on any drug active against one pole of the illness and shown not to make relapse to the other pole more likely.
- Lithium and olanzapine prevent relapse of mania, but are relatively less effective against depression.
- Lamotrigine is more effective against depression than mania in long-term treatment.
- Lithium reduces the risk of suicide.
- Valproate may be as effective as lithium in the prevention of relapse, but carbamazepine is less effective than lithium.
- When the risk of a severe depressive relapse is high, antidepressants to which patients have shown an acute treatment response may, if appropriate, be continued long term, in combination with a drug showing long-term antimanic efficacy.
- Discontinuation of long-term treatment is not indicated when there is good clinical control of the illness.
- Successful long-term management often appears to require combination treatment. At present, there is little to guide practice other than safety concerns and pragmatic outcomes in individual cases.
- There is no simple rule to determine whether treatment should be stopped during pregnancy: a clinical judgement is required, weighing the risks and benefits with the patient's preferences and past history.

fetal risk prior to conception, or withdrawing some or all medication prior to conception and reintroducing them either after the first trimester or immediately after birth. Slow-release formulations twice or more times daily can minimize high peak levels.

Patients prescribed lithium, valproate or carbamazepine during the first trimester should be told about prenatal diagnosis and offered maternal α-fetoprotein screening and a high-resolution ultrasound scan at 16–18 weeks' gestation. Folate supplementation is advised for all pregnant women and may reduce the increased risk of neural tube deficits associated with carbamazepine and valproate.

Childbirth increases the risk of subsequent early manic and depressive relapse and is a reason for increased clinical vigilance on the part of patients, carers and clinicians.

Key references

Altshuler L, Kiriakos L, Calcagno J et al. The impact of antidepressant discontinuation versus antidepressant continuation on 1-year risk for relapse of bipolar depression: a retrospective chart review. *J Clin Psychiatry* 2001;62(8):612–16.

Austin MP, Mitchell PB. Use of psychotropic medications in breast-feeding women: acute and prophylactic treatment. *Aust N Z J Psychiatry* 1998;32(6):778–84.

Buse JB. Metabolic side effects of antipsychotics: focus on hyperglycemia and diabetes. *J Clin Psychiatry* 2002;63(Suppl 4):37–41.

Cohen LS, Friedman JM, Jefferson JW et al. A re-evaluation of risk of in utero exposure to lithium. *JAMA* 1994;271(2):146–50.

Geddes JR, Carney SM, Davies C et al. Relapse prevention with antidepressant drug treatment in depressive disorders. *Lancet* 2003;361 :643–51.

Goodwin FK, Fireman B, Simon GE et al. Suicide risk in bipolar disorder during treatment with lithium and divalproex. *JAMA* 2003;290(11): 1467–73.

Goodwin GM. Recurrence of mania after lithium withdrawal. Implications for the use of lithium in the treatment of bipolar affective disorder. *Br J Psychiatry* 1994;164(2):149–52.

Greil W, Ludwig-Mayerhofer W, Erazo N et al. Lithium versus carbamazepine in the maintenance treatment of bipolar disorders – a randomised study. *J Affect Disord* 1997;43(2):151–61.

Okuma T, Kishimoto A. A history of investigation on the mood stabilizing effect of carbamazepine in Japan. *Psychiatry Clin Neurosci* 1998;52(1):3–12.

Prien RF, Kupfer DJ, Mansky PA et al. Drug therapy in the prevention of recurrences in unipolar and bipolar affective disorders. Report of the NIMH Collaborative Study Group comparing lithium carbonate, imipramine, and a lithium carbonate-imipramine combination. *Arch Gen Psychiatry* 1984;41(11):1096–104.

Smith S. Effects of antipsychotics on sexual and endocrine function in women: implications for clinical practice. *J Clin Psychopharmacol* 2003;23(3 Suppl 1):S27–32.

TABLE 7.1

Medicines used for long-term treatment

Additional information about medicines
For newer agents (the atypical antipsychotics), clinicians should refer to
company data sheets and emerging evidence. Unexpected adverse effects in
bipolar patients should be reported to the relevant licensing authority. There is
much accumulated experience to guide the use of lithium, but it is potentially

	Lithium	Valproate
Significant contraindications	• Renal impairment • Complicated fluid or salt balance • Acute myocardial infarction • Myasthenia gravis • Pregnancy	• Impairment of liver function • Blood dyscrasia

Drug interactions	• Diuretics
	• NSAIDs
	• Carbamazepine
	• Calcium channel blockers
	• ACE inhibitors
	• Metronidazole
	• Neuroleptics
		• Inhibits hepatic metabolism
		• Increases levels of
		  – Aspirin
		  – Anticoagulants
		  – Fatty acids
		  – Lamotrogine
		  – Ammonia

toxic and litigation is possible if accepted procedures are not followed. Experience with anticonvulsants in bipolar patients is growing, but is already extensive in patients with epilepsy. If in doubt, consult data sheets or individual manufacturers for latest safety information.

Carbamazepine	Lamotrigine
• Impairment of cardiac, renal or liver function • Prior hematologic dyscrasia	• Impairment of liver function • Renal impairment

• Induces P450
• Reduces levels of
  – Antipsychotics
  – Lamotrigine
  – Oral contraceptives
  – Many others
• Level of carbamazepine may be increased when P450 blocked by:
  – Fluoxetine
  – Valproate
  – Histamine H_2 blockers
  – Erythromycin
  – Isoniazid
  – Propoxiphene
  – Calcium channel blockers
• Carbamazepine + lithium may result in a rash
	• Valproate reduces metabolism, so it is necessary to halve dose of lamotrigine
	• Caution when using with carbamazepine
	  – double doses may be required but side effects may be increased

(CONTINUED)

TABLE 7.1 (CONTINUED)

	Lithium	Valproate

Most common adverse effects	• Gastrointestinal irritation
	• Sedation
	• Tremor
	• Other important effects:
	  – Weight gain
	  – Edema
	  – Acne
	  – Psoriasis
	  – Polyuria
	  – Polydipsia
		• Tremor
		• Dizziness
		• Sedation
		• Nausea/vomiting
		• Gastrointestinal pain
		• Headache
		• Elevated LFTs

Most worrisome adverse effects	• Acute intoxication:
	  – Seizure
	  – Coma
	  – Death
	• Intoxication sequelae:
	  – Renal
	  – Cardiac
	  – Central nervous system
	• At therapeutic levels:
	  – Thyroid inhibition
	  – Renal dysfunction
	  – Arrhythmias
	  – Teratogenicity
		• Marrow suppression
		• Thrombocytopenia
		• Prolongation of coagulation time
		• Pancreatitis
		• Hair loss
		• Weight gain
		• Teratogenicity

Carbamazepine	Lamotrigine
• Dizziness	• Dizziness
• Sedation	• Ataxia
• Unsteady gait	• Sedation
• Incoordination	• Insomnia
• Cognitive impairment	• Nausea/vomiting
• Blurred vision/diplopia	
• Elevated LFTs	
• Gastrointestinal	
– Nausea	
– Anorexia	
– Pain	
• Aplastic anemia	• Stevens–Johnson syndrome
• Agranulocytosis	• Other important effects:
• Thrombocytopenia	– Rash
• Hepatitis	– Blurred vision/diplopia
• Skin adverse effects:	– Esophagitis
– Rash (pruritic, erythematous)	
– Erythema multiforme or nodosum	
– Toxic epidermal necrolysis	
– Stevens–Johnson syndrome	
• Hyponatremia	
• Altered thyroid function	
• Edema	
• Arrhythmia, AV block	
• Alopecia	
• SLE	
• Potential teratogen	

(CONTINUED)

TABLE 7.1 (CONTINUED)

	Lithium	Valproate
Initiating long-term treatment	*Pretreatment assessments* • FBC • Electrolytes • Thyroid function tests • Creatinine • Urinalysis • ECG if clinically indicated *Initial dose regimen* 400 mg at night then titrate to the highest well-tolerated dose *Usual maintenance dose* 800–1200 mg, but lower in the elderly	*Pretreatment assessments* • FBC • Platelets • LFTs *Initial dose regimen* 250–500 mg twice daily Consider single dose at night *Alternative rapid titration* Day 1: single dose 20 mg/kg; day 2–4: continue split twice daily Target level > 80 µg/mL *During titration* consider serum valproate levels Usual maintenance dose 1250 mg/day or more
Follow-up laboratory tests	• Serum lithium 3-monthly and every 12 months or when clinically indicated: • Thyroid function tests • Creatinine • Urinalysis • FBC (expect neutrophilia)	• FBC and LFTs every 6–12 months or if clinically indicated

Carbamazepine	Lamotrigine
Pretreatment assessments	***Pretreatment assessments***
• FBC	• No laboratory tests required
• Platelets	***Initial dose regimen***
• LFTs	25 mg/day for 2 weeks, then
• Urinalysis	50 mg/day for 2 weeks, then
Initial dose regimen	increase each week by
400 mg at night	100 mg to usual maintenance
Titrate to clinical response	dose
(not to specific serum level)	***During titration:*** no laboratory
over 7–14 days	tests required
Usual maintenance dose	***Usual maintenance dose***
800 mg or more	200–400 mg/day
	If added to valproate, halve
	doses
	If added to carbamazepine,
	double doses (note that side
	effects may increase)
• Consider regular FBC and LFTs	Potentially useful (especially
	if lamotrigine is given
	concurrently with drug
	which alters metabolism)
	• Serum levels
	• LFTs

(CONTINUED)

TABLE 7.1 (CONTINUED)

	Lithium	Valproate
Points to cover in patient education	*Expect (one or more)* • Mild tremor • Thirst • Gastrointestinal irritation • Sedation *Report to doctor* • Moderate tremor • Slurred speech • Muscle twitching • Change in fluid balance • Memory impairment • Rash • Edema *Discuss* • Laboratory rationale • Weight control • Importance of sodium • Potential teratogenicity	*Expect* • Sedation • Tremor • Gastrointestinal symptoms *Report to doctor* • Easy bruising • Abdominal swelling • Rash • Jaundice • Edema (facial) *Discuss* • Weight control program • Common drug interactions • Potential teratogenicity • Use of vitamins/minerals (folate, selenium, zinc)

ACE, angiotensin-converting enzyme; FBC, full blood count; LFTs, liver function tests; NSAID, non-steroidal anti-inflammatory drug; SLE, systemic lupus erythematosus.

Carbamazepine	Lamotrigine
Expect	*Expect (transiently)*
• Sedation	• Insomnia/sedation
• Gastrointestinal symptoms	• Nausea
• Lightheadedness	• Dizziness
Report to doctor	*Report to doctor*
• Rash	• Rash
• Jaundice	• Easy bruising
• Incordination	• Abdominal swelling
• Irregular heartbeat	• Jaundice
• Facial edema	• Edema (facial)
Discuss	*Discuss*
• Importance of weight control program	• Common drug interactions
• Common drug interactions	• Use of vitamins/minerals (folate, selenium, zinc)
• Potential teratogenicity	
• Use of vitamins/minerals (folate, selenium, zinc)	

The foregoing chapters have painted a broad outline of the facts about bipolar disorder: its nature as a clinical problem, our attempts to classify it and understand the causes, and most importantly how we think it should best be treated. We hope that we have made the case for a scientific approach to psychiatry based on what has worked for other medical problems. We believe that this approach is starting to work for bipolar disorder too.

The discoveries that we expect will make a major difference in the coming years fall under three headings: genetics, neuroscience and treatment trials. We think they may change practice for the better, and so we hope patients and clinicians will support efforts to get the clinical work done. Making a case for progress may seem superfluous, but over-zealous ethical rule-making on the one hand, and an anti-science populism on the other, threaten research in all the areas that we believe will be most important for bipolar disorder, especially in Europe.

Genetics

Psychiatric geneticists have perhaps for too long promised too much and delivered very little. The Human Genome Project and the advances in technology that it has stimulated mean we do now stand on the threshold of knowing the molecular genetic associations of bipolar disorder. These associations are likely to inform our understanding of the etiology at every possible level. At its simplest, this could transform diagnosis because we will quickly see how far our phenotypic subtypes are reflected in genetic variation.

Genetic variation may also operate to modify environmental effects and treatment. Thus, pharmacogenetics may come to dominate how we choose between different pharmacological and non-pharmacological treatments, because some genotypes may favor a particular response to treatment more than others. We expect that the heterogeneity of response, which we can now simply witness, will be illuminated by genotyping. It will therefore inform how we select the most effective management plan for individual patients. The only threat to this kind of development will be if the numbers of genes involved are very large and individual genetic effects very small. We shall see.

Neuroscience

Neuroscience offers an integrated and essentially singular view of how the brain works, although it draws on the expertise of traditionally separate disciplines. Advances in cognitive psychology, psychopharmacology, brain imaging and cell biology are highly likely to change our understanding of what underlies mood and emotion in health. It seems inevitable that this understanding will also break down the current conceptual barriers to understanding psychiatric disease. This will be particularly important if we can identify the functional pathology of bipolar disorder. It may transform how we define outcomes in treatment studies and our understanding of how treatments work. Current strategies emphasize the treatment and prevention of syndromal relapse. Disabling aspects of long-term outcome, such as chronic depressive symptoms or enduring neurocognitive impairment, may be more important future therapeutic targets.

Improvements in treatment

Finally, we wish to see improvements in treatment. We have emphasized how care can be enhanced by structured psychological interventions and we expect to see further modest, but important, progress in this direction. However, bipolar disorder is a strongly biologically determined disease and we hope to see more effective use of drugs in the coming years.

Cancer chemotherapy has been transformed in the last 40 years not by magic bullets (although they would always be welcome), but by successful combination therapy with drugs that, individually, are ineffective and/or toxic. Clinical trials have established the efficacy and tolerability of the effective combination regimens.

Those of us with an interest in mood disorder may do psychiatry in general a favor by showing how this approach can also work for us. We already know that combination treatments are what we use in practice, yet we still await the results of the first randomized trials to prove that they are truly effective.

In conclusion, we have written this book at a time when something approaching a consensus has emerged among clinicians treating bipolar disorder. The accumulation of new evidence – the fast facts provided here – has made this possible. Consensus implies agreeing on what we know and also, sometimes more interestingly, on what we need to know. As we hope to have made plain, there are no grounds for complacency, but the research agenda is an exciting one. Only a commitment to clinical research in psychiatry from funding agencies, health services, clinicians and patients will deliver the knowledge we need for innovation and improvement.

Key references

Blumberg HP, Leung HC, Skudlarski P et al. A functional magnetic resonance imaging study of bipolar disorder: state- and trait-related dysfunction in ventral prefrontal cortices. *Arch Gen Psychiatry* 2003;60(6):601–9.

Flint J. Animal models of anxiety and their molecular dissection. *Semin Cell Dev Biol* 2003;14(1):37–42.

Geddes J, Goodwin G. Bipolar disorder: clinical uncertainty, evidence-based medicine and large-scale randomised trials. *Br J Psychiatry* 2001;41(suppl):s191–4.

Hyman SE. Goals for research on bipolar disorder: the view from NIMH. *Biol Psychiatry* 2000;48(6):436–41.

Insel TR, Charney DS. Research on major depression: strategies and priorities. *JAMA* 2003;289(23):3167–8.

Watson JD. Genes and politics. *J Mol Med* 1997;75(9):624–36.

Useful resources

American Psychiatric
Association (APA)
www.psych.org/

American Psychological
Association
www.apa.org/

Bipolar Significant Others (BPSO)
http://www.bpso.org/

British Association for
Psychopharmacology
www.bap.org.uk/

Child and Adolescent Bipolar
Foundation
www.bpkids.org/

Depression and Bipolar Support
Alliance (DBSA)
US patient organisation with
many useful links
www.dbsalliance.org/index.html

Electronic Medicines
Compendium
List of all licensed medications
available in the UK
www.medicines.org.uk/

Harvard Bipolar Research Program
For information on research and
treatment, including the STEP-BD
program, and many useful links
www.manicdepressive.org/

Manic Depression Fellowship
UK patient organisation
www.mdf.org.uk/

Medscape
A large US database linked to
other useful medical databases
psychiatry.medscape.com/

National Alliance for the
Mentally Ill
www.nami.org

National electronic Library for
Mental Health
One of the specialist libraries
accessible at the National
electronic Library for Health
website
www.nelh.nhs.uk/

Netdoctor
Features information and the
latest news on depression,
discussion forums and chatrooms,
support services and an 'ask the
expert' service where a question
can be put to an expert panel.
www.depression.netdoctor.co.uk/

Society for Manic Depression
www.societymd.org/index.html

Pendulum Resources
An on-line support group for
manic-depressives.
www.pendulum.org/

Disclosure

The authors are conscious of the current controversies about conflict of interest in scientific and especially medical writing. We regard ourselves as holding independent opinions and we have expressed them as honestly as we can in this book. However, like most, if not all, responsible adults in professional positions, we have potential conflicts of interest. By conflicts of interest we mean relationships, allegiances or hostilities to particular groups, organizations or interests, which could excessively influence our judgements or actions. The issue is obviously most sensitive when such interests are private and/or may result in personal gain. We have identified a hierarchy of such possible interests in declaring ours.

Guy Goodwin

- Neither I nor my family hold patents or inventions or own part of any company (including shares) with interests in the area of psychopharmacology.
- I have never accepted a personal retainer from any company with an interest in psychopharmacology.
- I have acted within the last year as a paid consultant to Bristol-Myers Squibb, Lundbeck, Pfizer, GlaxoSmithKline and AstraZeneca. I have also advised Lilly and Janssen in the past.
- I have acted as an expert witness for Pfizer.
- I hold an agreement with Sanofi to supply Depakote for an independent clinical trial.
- I am not a formal member of the speakers' bureau for any company.
- I have accepted many paid speaking engagements in industry-supported symposia.
- I have occasionally accepted travel or hospitality unrelated to a speaking engagement from a pharmaceutical company.
- My primary employment is with Oxford University and the National Health Service in England.

Gary Sachs

- My family has a substantial ownership interest in Concordant Raters Systems, LLC. I hold patent on systems tools invented for training and monitoring raters in the using of rating scales in clinical research studies.

- Neither I nor my family have any other patents or inventions nor own any company with interests in the area of psychopharmacology.
- I have never accepted a personal retainer from any company with an interest in psychopharmacology.
- I have acted within the past year as a paid advisory board member or consultant to Abbott Laboratories, AstraZeneca, Bristol-Myers Squibb, Pfizer, GlaxoSmithKline, Lilly and Janssen. In the past, I have also advised Elan, Sanofi and Solvay.
- I currently conduct research studies funded by the National Institute of Mental Health, Abbott and Janssen.
- I hold agreements with Abbott and GlaxoSmithKline to supply medication for National Institute of Mental Health sponsored research projects.
- I am a member of the speakers' bureau or have given lectures or symposia sponsored by Abbott, AstraZeneca, Bristol-Myers Squibb, GlaxoSmithKline, Lilly, OrthoMcNeil.
- My primary employment is with Massachusetts General Hospital and Harvard University in the USA.

Appendix: Generic and brand names of drugs

Generic names	US brand names	UK brand names
Drugs used in the treatment of patients with bipolar disorder		
Aripiprazole	Abilify	Not yet available
Bupropion	Wellbutrin Zyban	Zyban
Carbamazepine	Atretol Carbatrol Epitol Tegretol	Teril Retard Tegretol
Chlorpromazine	Thorazine	Largactil
Citalopram	Celexa	Cipramil
Clonazepam	Klonopin	Rivotril
Clozapine	Clozaril	Clozaril
Escitalopram	Lexapro	Cipralex
Fluoxetine	Prozac	Prozac
Fluvoxamine	Luvox	Faverin
Gabapentin	Neurontil	Neurontin
Haloperidol	Haldol	Dozic Haldol Serenace
Lamotrigine	Lamictal	Lamictal
Lithium (carbonate/citrate)	Eskalith Eskalith CR Lithobid	Camcolit Li-liquid Liskonum Priadel
Lorazepam	Ativan	Ativan
Moclobemide	–	Manerix
Olanzapine	Zyprexa	Zyprexa
Oxcarbazepine	Trileptal	Trileptal
Paroxetine	Paxil	Seroxat
Phenelzine	Nardil	Nardil
Quetiapine	Seroquel	Seroquel

Generic names	US brand names	UK brand names
Risperidone	Risperdal	Risperdal
Sertraline	Zoloft	Lustral
Trancylpromine	Parnate	Parnate
Valproate	Depakene Depakote	Depakote
Ziprasidone	Geodon	Not available in UK
Other drugs referred to in text		
Amphetamine	Adderal Dexedrine Focalin	Dexedrine
Levodopa	Atamet Sinemet	Madopar Sinemet
Topiramate	Topamax	Topamax

Index

acute treatment 17, 68
  see also short-term
adrenocorticotropic hormone 5
adverse effects
  carbamazepine 83
  lamotrigine 83
  lithium 82
  valproate 82
advice to patients 53–4
affective disorder 7
affective experience 4
akathisia 5, 60
alcohol misuse 17, 18, 42, 49,
  53, 77
American Psychiatric
  Association 4, 61
amphetamine 24, 35, 95
anticonvulsants 65, 66, 71,
  73–4
  see also valproate; and others
  by name
antidepressants 16, 17, 18, 32,
  56, 63–5, 66, 74–5, 78
  see also MAOIs; SSRIs; and
  others by name
antimanic drugs 4, 24, 58, 64,
  67, 68, 78
antipsychotic drugs 4, 5, 6, 24,
  48, 56, 58–60, 61, 62, 64,
  65, 67, 68, 69, 74, 75, 76, 77
  see also chlorpromazine;
  olanzapine; and others by
  name
anti-science populism 88
anxiety 4, 27
anxiety-related disorders 16, 18
aripiprazole 57, 59, 68, 77, 95
attention 4
Axis I 4, 18
Axis II 4, 18

basal ganglia 5
benzodiazepines 48, 56, 62, 68
biological rhythms 28
bipolar I disorder 4, 13, 14,
  16, 18, 25, 27, 28, 29, 32,
  33, 35, 54, 55, 64, 71, 75
bipolar II disorder 4, 13, 14,
  16, 18, 33, 35, 75

bipolar spectrum disorder 18,
  19, 32, 68
British Association for
  Psychopharmacology (BAP)
  55, 56, 63, 64, 71, 72
bupropion 65, 95

carbamazepine 56, 57, 60–1,
  66, 72, 73, 75, 78, 81, 83,
  85, 87, 95,
  in pregnancy 77, 78–9
cell biology 89
children see young patients
chlorpromazine 4, 57, 58, 95
chronic symptoms 55
citalopram/escitalopram 65, 95
clonazepam 58, 95
clozapine 57, 74, 77, 95
cognitive–behavior therapy
  (CBT) 4, 51–3, 64, 72
cognitive impairment 4, 8,
  61
cognitive psychology 89
combination treatment 56,
  61–2, 68, 69, 75–6, 78,
  89–90
commitment to clinical
  research 90
communication with
  patients 47
comorbidity 16–17, 18, 42
compassionate relationship
  with patient 45
compliance/adherence to
  medicines 17, 49, 51, 52, 53,
  61, 72, 76, 77
concentration, difficulty in 15
contraindications
  carbamazepine 81
  lamotrigine 81
  lithium 80
  valproate 80
cortical lesions 17
corticosteroids 17
corticotropin 26
corticotropin-releasing
  hormone 5
cortisol 5, 24, 27, 29
counseling 4

creative artists as sufferers
  39–42, 45
  artists 41
  composers 41
  poets 40–1
  writers 40
Cushing's disease 26, 27
cyclothymia 14

death, fear of 15
delusions 5, 12
dementia praecox 7
depression 4, 7, 13, 14, 16, 18,
  22, 23, 25–6, 27, 32, 37, 42,
  45, 62, 72
  refractory 28, 68
  short-term treatments 63–8,
  69
  see also major depression
despair 7
dexamethasone 26
  suppression test (DST) 26
diabetes (type 2) 76
diagnosis 4, 11–19, 32, 34, 35,
  36, 54, 56, 64, 72, 88
  see also differential diagnosis
differential diagnosis 17
diffusion tensor imaging 30
discontinuation of long-term
  treatment 76, 77, 78
dopamine 4, 5, 24–5, 29,
  58–9, 77
dopamine hypothesis 24
drug absorption 5
drug company data sheets 80
drug interactions
  carbamazepine 81
  lamotrigine 81
  lithium 80
  valproate 80
drug metabolism 5
drug-induced psychosis 17
DSM-IV 4, 6, 11–15, 17, 18,
  32, 33, 35
dystonic reactions 5, 60

elation 4, 11, 14
electroconvulsive therapy
  (ECT) 5, 56, 63, 64, 66, 69

endocrine function 26–7
abnormalities 27–8
endogenous origins 5
enhanced case 47–54
epidemiology 32–5
ethical rule-making,
over-zealous 88
etiology 14, 20–31, 88
euphoria 7, 13, 14, 27, 29, 37
euthymia 16, 23, 24, 26, 29,
55, 72
executive function 4
exogenous origins 5
expansiveness 12, 13
extrapyramidal side effects
(EPS) 5, 57, 59, 60, 61, 62,
68, 76, 77

family and friends 47, 49, 52
fatigue 15
first-degree relatives 14, 18, 21
see also heritability
fluoxetine 63, 65, 67, 95
fluvoxamine 65, 95
follow-up laboratory tests
carbamazepine 85
lamotrigine 85
lithium 84
valproate 84
functional neuropathology
28–9
future discoveries expected
genetics 88–9
neuroscience 89
treatment trials 89–90
future studies 9

gabapentin 61, 71, 95
gait disturbance 5
gastrointestinal side effects 61
generalized anxiety disorder 16
genetic variation 88
genetics of bipolar disorder see
heritability; neurobiology
genotyping and management
planning 89
glucocorticoids 26
guilt 15

hallucinations 5, 12
haloperidol 57, 60, 61, 68,
95
heritability 14, 20–2, 29, 88–9
history of bipolar disorder 7

hospital admission 11, 12, 29,
32, 55, 56, 63
Human Genome Project 88
hyperactivity 34–5
hyperprolactinemia 77
hypersomnia 14, 15
hyperthyroidism 12, 27
hypomania 4, 5, 13, 16, 17,
18, 27, 32, 33, 35, 42, 45
hypothalamic–pituitary–adrenal
(HPA) axis 5, 23, 26, 29
hypothalamus 5, 25, 26
hypothyroidism 16, 27

imipramine 63, 74
impaired function 5, 11, 12,
13, 14, 18
indecisiveness 15
initiating treatment
carbamazepine 85
lamotrigine 85
lithium 84
valproate 84
insomnia 15
interpersonal therapy (IPT) 64
irritability 5, 12, 14

knowledge/psychoeducation
47–8, 53
Kraepelin, Emil 7–8

lamotrigine 61, 64, 65, 66, 69,
72, 73–4, 77, 78, 81, 83, 85,
87, 95
levodopa 17, 95
lithium 25, 27, 56, 57, 58,
60–1, 62, 64, 65, 66, 68, 69,
71, 72, 73, 75, 76, 78, 80,
82, 84, 86, 95
in pregnancy 77, 78–9
long-term treatments 61,
71–87
adverse effects 76–7
anticonvulsants 73–4
antidepressants 74
antipsychotics 74–5
combination therapy 72, 75–6
discontinuation 76
lithium 71, 72, 73
pregnancy and childbirth
77–9
treatment scheme 72
lorazepam 58, 95
loss of interest/pleasure 15

magnetic resonance imaging
(MRI) 26
maintenance treatment 56,
64, 72
major/severe depression 4, 5,
6, 13, 14, 18, 21, 26, 32, 35
mania 4, 5, 6, 7, 11–13,
14, 16, 18, 22, 23, 24–5,
26, 27, 29, 32, 37, 38, 39,
45, 67
short-term treatments 55–63
see also secondary mania
melancholia 7
memory 4, 5, 66
mixed states 13–14, 16, 74
short-term treatments 55–63
moclobemide 65, 95
molecular genetics 88
monoamine oxidase inhibitors
(MAOIs) 65
mood chart 49, 50
mood depression 7, 15, 50
mood disturbances/disorder
4, 6, 12, 22, 23, 26,
27, 28, 29, 32, 35, 45,
89–90
mood elevation 5, 7, 12, 13,
14, 18, 24, 35, 50
mood stabilizers 66, 71,
73, 78
mood variation 14
morbidity 33
multiple sclerosis 17

neurobiology 8, 21, 23–4, 29,
88, 89
neuroimaging 29–30, 89
neuroleptics 4
neurotransmitters 4, 5, 23,
24, 28
see also dopamine; and
others by name
norepinephrine/noradrenaline
26, 28, 29
nurses 9

obsessive–compulsive disorder
16
olanzapine 57, 59–60, 61, 62,
65, 67, 68, 71, 72, 74, 77,
78, 95
outpatient supervision 72
overactivity 12, 13
oxcarbazepine 57, 61, 95